Hispanic Families at Risk

Ronald J. Angel · Jacqueline L. Angel

Hispanic Families at Risk

The New Economy, Work, and the Welfare State

Springer

Ronald J. Angel
Department of Sociology
University of Texas, Austin
1 University Station
Austin TX 78712
Box A 1700
USA
rangel@austin.utexas.edu

Jacqueline L. Angel
Department of Sociology
University of Texas, Austin
1 University Station
Austin TX 78712
Box A 1700
USA
jangel@mail.utexas.edu

ISBN 978-1-4419-0473-7 e-ISBN 978-1-4419-0474-4
DOI 10.1007/978-1-4419-0474-4
Springer Dordrecht Heidelberg London New York

Library of Congress Control Number: 2009927011

Printed on acid-free paper

Springer is part of Springer Science+Business Media (www.springer.com)

Preface: The Hispanic Labor Force and the Employment-Based Welfare State

Unlike the nations of Europe that have only recently begun to accept the fact that immigration is an integral part of their cultural and social realities, the United States has always embraced its identity as a nation of immigrants, even if newer arrivals have not always been welcomed with open arms or treated with respect by those who came earlier. For the immigrants from Europe who came to America in the nineteenth and early twentieth centuries, the United States promised the real possibility of economic success and upward social mobility. In a rapidly growing nation with many entry-level jobs, the first rung on the ladder of economic progress was relatively easy to reach. Even for eastern and southern Europeans the fact of racial similarity made assimilation relatively easy and after a few generations hardly any notable distinctions among national origin groups remained. As Richard Alba noted nearly 20 years ago, over time European immigrants lost their unique cultural identities and outward markers and evolved a true "European American" ethnic identity (Alba 1990). For these groups the new country was truly a melting pot and the retention of any aspect of one's original cultural identity was a matter of choice that remained mostly symbolic.

For more recent immigrants from other parts of the world, the incorporation experience has been far different. During the latter part of the twentieth and the beginning of the twenty-first centuries, the vast majority of immigrants have come from Asia and Latin America (He 2002). Although some of these new immigrants, especially those with advanced technical skills, have done quite well, others, and especially those with little human capital, have not (Duncan and Trejo 2005; Portes et al. 2005; Portes and Rumbaut 2001; Portes and Zhou 1993; Telles and Ortiz 2008). Although immigration is not the core focus of this book, we are forced to deal with the issue of immigration because of its salience for the Hispanic, and especially the Mexican-origin population. The issue of the incorporation of immigrants into the economic mainstream also serves as a way of framing the problem of low levels of work-related benefits, including retirement plans and group health insurance coverage, among Hispanics.

Although certain Mexican Americans have been citizens since the United States annexed the northern part of Mexico in 1848, even for segments of this group the economic incorporation process is not complete and questions remain as to whether it ever will be. For large segments of the Mexican-origin population, middle-class economic security remains elusive even after generations. As a result, many Mexican-origin youth seem to have abandoned the hope for middle-class success and have adopted a behavioral orientation that minimizes the value of education and reflects a marginalized social identity (Espinosa and Ochoa 1986; Matute-Bianchi 1986; Portes and Rumbaut 2001; Romo and Falbo 1996; Suárez-Orozco and Suárez-Orozco 1995). Faced with what appear to be insurmountable barriers to moving ahead, certain individuals turn their back on middle-class culture and embrace a counterproductive life in gangs and on the street (Hagan and Peterson 1995). Educational levels in the Mexican-origin population remain shockingly low and high school dropout rates far exceed those of other groups (Matute-Bianchi 1986; Romo and Falbo 1996). Even if they remain in school, Mexican-origin students perform less well than other students (Portes 1999).

The economic and social situation of the Mexican-origin population, then, is complex and reflects factors related to immigration, low educational levels, and occupational disadvantage (Duncan and Trejo 2005; Portes and Rumbaut 1996; Telles and Ortiz 2008). Sociologists and others who study immigration have employed the phrase "segmented assimilation" to characterize the situation in which some segments of the population fail to move ahead economically, occupationally, or socially. The concept of segmented assimilation serves to draw attention to the fact that for certain individuals, upward mobility and economic success are not inevitable, and it motivates us to ask what the reasons for this blocked assimilation might be. The notion that a group consists of segments or strata with different cultural, social, and personal characteristics that determine their chances of upward mobility provides a theoretical and empirical means of understanding why some Mexican-origin families have become members of the middle class while others have not.

Among successful Mexican-origin families, one finds those headed by doctors, lawyers, professors, and well-paid professionals of all sorts. These families own homes, purchase stocks and bonds, and participate in employment-based retirement and health insurance plans. Among the unsuccessful, one finds families that never made the transition from an economically marginalized status to the middle class. These families, some of whom consist of old-stock Mexican Americans, never succeeded in making the transition out of the lower classes and many become permanent members of a stigmatized underclass. In this book we define "success" as entry into the American middle class, at least economically. In addition to an adequate income, though, being middle class implies the adoption of certain norms that include a high value on education and the desire to see one's children do better than oneself. A central goal of most families is to assure that their children receive a good education and obtain a good job. For new arrivals the objective is upward mobility and even greater success for the second and subsequent generations. Such success, of course, depends on an adequate income. With a good income one can save money, buy a home, educate one's children, take vacations, help others in need, and do much more. Successful families make up successful communities with collective economic and social assets and resources that can be used to start businesses, further the ambitions of individuals, or deal with the setbacks experienced by any one family.

The Absence of Employment Benefits

As central as income and wealth are to the determination of a family's security and long-term prospects, though, employment-based benefits are essential. Indeed, the very definition of a good job or a profession includes not only an adequate income but also retirement and health benefits. Since at least World War II, retirement and health benefits have become a routine aspect of professional occupations and they have become a central component of negotiations between management and labor (Asher and Stephenson 1990; Quadagno 2005; Weir et al. 1988). In order to attract and retain highly trained and productive employees, employers must offer attractive benefit packages. Today even for middle-class workers, employment-based benefits are becoming less generous. As health-care costs soar, so does the cost of health insurance and many employers find it necessary to shift a greater portion of the cost onto employees who sometimes find that they cannot afford the premiums. Defined benefit retirement plans that insure a worker a predictable income for life are being replaced by defined contribution plans that place the responsibility for insuring sufficient retirement income on the employee (Munnell and Sundén 2004). The economic crisis that began in 2008 means those even large employers must renegotiate labor contracts and make financial cutbacks that threaten the generosity of benefit plans even further.

For many middle-class Americans, then, the income and health-care security that came to define a good job after World War II is eroding. For those individuals and families who never made it into the middle class, including a large segment of the Hispanic population, this erosion of benefits is less relevant. For those who have traditionally worked in jobs that do not offer benefits there is little to lose. Individuals in lower tier service sector jobs and the chronically unemployed never have been able to save for retirement or future consumption, nor has health insurance ever been part of the equation. The new benefit insecurity that is unsettling segments of the middle class has been business as usual for poor Hispanic families. The employment-based welfare state in the United States stands in stark contrast to that of other developed nations in which universal health care and other benefits are provided as public goods.

The Social Safety Net Across the Life Course

In the absence of employment benefits, one must rely on publicly funded programs such as Medicaid and the State Children's Health Insurance Plan (SCHIP) for health care. For non-disabled childless adults, public health coverage is basically nonexistent. Without a retirement plan, one must rely on personal savings, the equity in one's home, or other assets to finance one's final years. A job that does not offer a retirement plan, though, is not likely to pay enough to allow a person to save much at all. The lack of benefits is part of a cycle of poverty that can be truly vicious and low-wage workers often find themselves trapped in an economic morass from which families and entire communities cannot escape.

In the following chapters we examine the employment-based benefit system that defines the US welfare state and identify those barriers that many Hispanic and especially Mexican-origin families face in gaining access to such benefits. When we conceived of this book project, our intention was to focus on the Mexican-origin population that we have been studying for 30 years. Mexican-origin individuals, who define their ethnic origin or ancestors as "Mexican," make up over 60% of the Hispanic population and are the least likely of any group to have health insurance or retirement plans. The lack of such benefits accompanies the well-documented disadvantages experienced by the Mexican-origin population in terms of education, income, and wealth. The fact that a large fraction of the Mexican-origin population has little access to such benefits explains a large fraction of the economic insecurity of Hispanics as a whole.

Unfortunately, much governmental and other data available related to employment and work-related benefits that include Mexican-origin samples report results in terms of a combined Hispanic category. Rather than restrict our presentation to the data we and others have collected on the Mexican-origin population, we employ the wider range of information related to Hispanics. Comparisons of analyses based on the Mexican-origin population alone and those based on the combined Hispanic population reveal similar patterns, largely because of the fact that in representative samples the Mexican-origin segment dominates and its contribution to aggregate patterns is clearly obvious. In what follows, then, when we use the term Hispanic we are referring to data that combine Mexican-origin individuals and other Hispanics. When we can, we focus on the Mexican-origin population and use the term Mexican-origin.

An Outline of the Following Chapters

Each of the chapters in this book focuses on a different dimension of the employment-based benefit system of the United States and its impact on the economic security and health-care access for the Hispanic population. Although we focus heavily on the Mexican-origin population, the implications of the problems we identify in an employment-based system of social welfare are relevant to other vulnerable groups. The study is in the tradition of political and organizational sociology and reveals the fundamental weaknesses of the social welfare state in the United States relative to other developed nations. Our presentation takes a life-course perspective and examines the implications of low-wage employment and few or no benefits for the children of such workers, the workers themselves and their spouses, and the elderly.

In Chapter 1 we examine the nature of the employment-based social welfare state in the United States and its implications for the Mexican-origin population. We identify those structural sources of disadvantage associated with low levels of education and employment in sectors of the economy and in jobs in which benefits are not offered or offered at a cost that is prohibitive to low-wage workers. Although our discussion focuses on the Mexican-origin population, the structural barriers to benefits we identify also affect other groups.

In Chapter 2 we document the growth in the Hispanic population of the United States, of which the Mexican-origin population is the largest group. In this chapter we delve more deeply into the nature of employment among Mexican-origin workers including the economic sectors in which they find employment and the nature of the jobs they hold within sectors. As we demonstrate, Mexican-origin workers experience an occupational "ghettoization" in that they are disproportionately employed in sectors and jobs that do not offer benefits. This fact explains a large fraction of the Mexican-origin disadvantage.

In Chapter 3 we examine the effects of low levels of parental benefit coverage on children. Families with low incomes and no health insurance find themselves dependent on welfare, food stamps, housing assistance, as well as on Medicaid and the State Children's Health Insurance Program (SCHIP). Given the inadequacy of employment in terms of providing access to basic services, individuals in low-wage jobs, as well as the unemployed or underemployed, find themselves particularly dependent on publicly funded services. Yet many families that qualify for services on the basis of low family income do not participate in public programs and, consequently, many poor children do not receive the care they need (Centers for Medicare and Medicaid Services 2005). For parents at the economic margin, obtaining the services their children need is time consuming and can interfere with attempts to achieve economic security.

In Chapters 4 and 5 we investigate the ways in which gender affects health insurance coverage and the access to retirement plans. In Chapter 4 we examine employment patterns and benefit coverage among working-age males. In this chapter we document the fact that Mexican-origin males are more likely than other males to be employed in agriculture and the low-wage service sector in which benefit coverage is low. Even within sectors, though, Mexican-origin males are less likely than workers from other groups to have health or retirement coverage. The implications of inadequate retirement coverage are serious. Without the capacity to save and in the absence of an employer-based retirement plan, old-age income insecurity is almost inevitable. In addition, given the fact that there are almost no public sources of health care for nondisabled working-age males, the lack of employment-based health insurance represents a serious health risk.

In Chapter 5 we examine the access to benefits among Mexican-origin women under the age of 65. For women, marriage has traditionally served as the source of income security as well as the major source of health-care coverage and retirement security. The male breadwinner model upon which Social Security and other programs are based defines the family as the core social institution for providing individual security and support. For minority women, including those of Mexican origin, marriage has never guaranteed income security or access to basic health care (Shuey and Willson 2008; Willson 2003). Those women with husbands employed in low-wage service sector jobs are at elevated risk of lacking health-care coverage and an adequate retirement income. Late-life divorce, widowhood, and low-wage jobs contribute to this high risk of retirement insecurity. Some women, of course, are employed and have access to such benefits through their own employment. For many women, including a large fraction of Mexican-origin women, neither marriage nor employment guarantees an adequate family income or benefits.

In Chapter 6 we turn our attention to the elderly and examine their retirement incomes and health insurance coverage. Given a lifetime of employment in low-wage jobs that did not provide benefits, many older Mexican-origin retirees find themselves in dire economic straits. Although Social Security and Medicare have greatly reduced the level of extreme poverty and improved health-care access among the elderly, those who have no private retirement income, few assets, and no supplemental Medigap insurance to pay the costs of health care not covered by Medicare face serious debt if they become ill (Jacoby et al. 2001). With low retirement incomes, often consisting of Social Security alone and with little accumulated wealth, these individuals have little ability to help younger generations.

In Chapter 7 we conclude the presentation with an examination of future policy directions and possible reforms to deal with the problems inherent in an employment-based retirement and health insurance system for low-wage Americans and summarize the unique vulnerabilities of Mexican-origin workers and families. The basic weaknesses of an employment-based system have become particularly clear during the recession that followed the subprime mortgage disaster. Even for those who have access to retirement plans, defined contribution plans are for the most part woefully underfunded and will not provide the income that a retired worker and his family will need. In addition, individuals in low-wage jobs often find themselves without health insurance just when they need it most. It is clear from our analysis that in the absence of universal publicly funded health care and in the absence of an adequate retirement income, a large fraction of the Mexican-origin population, along with large numbers of other low-income Americans, faces permanent exclusion from the American dream.

Acknowledgement

This book is a product of our active collaboration that began more than 20 years ago when we began our investigation of the sociology of health and well-being in the Hispanic population. Over the past couple of decades, we have benefited greatly from the valuable insights of numerous colleagues and graduate students especially during our years at The University of Texas at Austin. We have benefited from the intellectual insights of members of the Hispanic community in the United States and colleagues in Mexico and Latin America, all of which are reflected in the message of this work. Special thanks are due to Jennifer Karas Montez and Kate Chambers, both of whom provided valuable research assistance during the last year of this project. We are grateful for the financial support of the National Institute on Aging and the National Institute of Child Health and Human Development.

Contents

Chapter 1
Hispanic Workers and the Employment-Based Welfare State

Compared with other developed nations, federal and state governments in the United States play a relatively limited role in providing the full range of social services to citizens (Hicks 1999; Noble 1997; Weir et al. 1988). Unlike the citizens of Europe, Americans do not expect free higher education, state-mandated vacations, family allowances, or publicly funded health care. Those over the age of 65 years enjoy the protections of income support and universal health care through Social Security and Medicare, but for working-age adults no such universal programs exist. In the United States, retirement security and health insurance are primarily work-related benefits. Unfortunately, for many working Americans, and especially minority Americans, their jobs do not guarantee health-care coverage or a guaranteed retirement income. In the absence of work-related benefits, few options exist. Jobs that do not provide benefits are unlikely to pay well enough to allow an individual to save for retirement or to purchase a family health insurance plan in the private market. For low-wage workers, the vast majority of their income goes to daily consumption and the satisfaction of basic needs.

When work does not provide these essential social benefits, either because one is unemployed or because one's work is informal or does not offer coverage, serious hardship can result. In this chapter, we examine the structural sources of high levels of vulnerability in terms of health and retirement coverage among Hispanic workers, with a particular focus on those of Mexican origin. Although we focus on the Mexican-origin population because of its particularly serious lack of health and retirement coverage, the structural sources of benefit insecurity affect all low-wage Americans. We begin, then, with the observation that more than in any other developed nation, in the United States one's economic, retirement, and health security depend on the nature of one's employment. Individuals with good jobs not only receive adequate incomes but live secure in the knowledge that the health care their families' need will be paid for by employment-based health insurance, and they can be certain that their retirement years will be comfortable because of private retirement plans and Social Security. A good job allows one to save enough to pay for a child's education, to buy a home or help a child buy a home, or to start a business. Those whose jobs pay well can often retire early and enjoy a life of leisure, or they can change careers and engage in activities that express their generativity. Individuals with bad jobs, which by definition are those that not only pay poorly but do not

R.J. Angel, J.L. Angel, *Hispanic Families at Risk*, DOI 10.1007/978-1-4419-0474-4_1,

offer employee benefits, face multiple insecurities throughout life. They live with the risk of inadequate health care, and their ability to provide higher education to their children or to retire comfortably remains limited.

The core theme that we develop in this and subsequent chapters is that as a result of the employment-based social welfare state that has evolved in the United States, groups that suffer structured disadvantages in the labor force face serious handicaps in terms of other basic social supports. For these individuals and families, the social safety net is often seriously inadequate. As we document extensively, along with other vulnerable groups, the Mexican-origin population is disadvantaged in all areas. Before proceeding, though, we must clarify what we mean by the "welfare state" and review a bit of the history of the role of government in providing the basic necessities of a productive and dignified life to its citizens, as well as explain why the United States is unique among developed nations in the limited nature of its welfare state.

The Modern Welfare State

The modern welfare state is a fairly recent development that is often traced to Germany in the mid-nineteenth century when Otto Von Bismarck introduced sickness, accident, and old-age benefits as part of the attempt to counter the rise of socialism (Sigerist 1999). The welfare state as it has evolved since Bismarck's day insures the basic social rights of citizens. Social rights refer to more than political rights; the term refers to the right of citizens to the basic material and social requirements of a productive and dignified life, including education, employment, health care, housing, old-age security, and more. The concept of the all-inclusive welfare state that insures both political and social citizenship rights has been described as the end of a process of political and social evolution, perhaps best summarized by T. H. Marshall several decades ago (Marshall 1950). Marshall summarized the development of the welfare state in England in terms of three historical periods that make up what he saw as the consolidation of basic human rights. According to Marshall the process began in the eighteenth century when peasants became citizens and won guarantees of fundamental legal and civil rights. That period was followed in the nineteenth century by the extension of political rights to larger segments of the population, or at least the white male population. Finally, during the twentieth century the process reached maturity in terms of the welfare state in which social rights were recognized as basic.

As is apparent from the political debates surrounding welfare both in the United States and in Europe, not everyone believes that individuals have legitimate claims to social rights at public expense. Many political theorists strongly reject the proposition that material security is a right (Etzioni 1993, 1995, 2000; Mead 1986, 1997; Murray 1994, 1996, 1999, 2006). For communitarians, libertarians, and others on the right, social policy based on the concept of social rights not only is expensive but creates welfare dependency and contributes to the growth of an underclass. These critics believe that basic political rights, consisting primarily of protections from interference by others or the State in carrying out one's wishes, are the only basic rights. Material welfare is in effect a commodity that one can purchase on the open market to the extent that one is able but which one has no right to at public expense. The new welfare philosophy reflected in the new "third way" in Britain and elsewhere and the Personal Responsibility and Work Opportunity Reconciliation Act of 1996 in the United States emphasizes citizens' duties as well as rights. Central among these duties is the requirement that one seek and accept gainful employment (Dwyer 2004a; Giddens 1998). Critics on the left object to the concept of social rights for very different reasons. They see the focus on a minimal level of material well-being as an incomplete or partial solution to the problems of the working class that require more radical solutions (for a useful overview, see Dwyer 2004b).

Marshall's characterization of the welfare state is clearly idealistic and really can only be taken to reflect English social history. Nonetheless, Marshall's description of the process of the evolution of human rights in England reflects a fairly common belief in the developed world today that full citizenship and a dignified existence require more than just the right not to be detained without cause or denied the right to vote. Full citizenship also includes guaranteed access to affordable and adequate nutrition, shelter, education, and health care. For many Europeans, basic social rights have even come to include the right to several weeks of paid vacation. Obviously, for a large fraction of the world's population, the most basic political rights are not guaranteed and social rights remain a distant dream. Even in developed nations many individuals are not guaranteed the same social rights as others. Indigenous peoples and racial and ethnic minorities are among these groups. Resistance to social welfare for the poor has been influenced by racial prejudices both in the United States and in Britain (Dwyer 2004b; Quadagno 1994). This fact has given rise to a heated debate over multiculturalism and the collective rights of groups such as Native Americans, African-Americans, and Hispanics. These debates center on the special situations of groups that are culturally different and those that have been involuntarily incorporated through conquest or slavery. We will review this debate and its implications for minority Americans in Chapter 2.

US Exceptionalism: A Limited Welfare State

The specific nature of each nation's welfare state clearly reflects unique historical, economic, political, and cultural factors. Gøsta Esping-Andersen (1990) proposed a frequently cited typology that consists of three types of welfare states that reflect different histories of the nations to which they apply. The Social Democratic type, typified by Sweden, Norway, and Denmark, is characterized by comprehensive cradle-to-grave system of social supports financed by high taxes. The Conservative model, which is typical of central European states such as Austria, Belgium, France, Germany, and Italy, evolved along more corporatist or class-based lines with generous benefits closely tied to union membership and labor sector affiliations. Both of these types of welfare states insure universal health care and provide other social benefits such as family allowances, housing assistance, free higher education, and more. The third type of welfare state, which Esping-Andersen labels "Liberal," is typical of the United States, Australia, New Zealand, and Canada, countries that rely more on the market for basic social protections and minimizes the role of the government. In these countries, and especially in the United States, publicly funded programs tend to be means-tested and focused on the marginal members of society who lack the capacity to provide for themselves.

The meaning of the term "welfare," like the welfare state itself, is very different in Europe and the United States. In the United States, the term "welfare" refers to means-tested assistance for the poor and does not bring to mind basic citizenship rights. The term is commonly used pejoratively and gives rise to images of welfare cheats and individuals who choose not to work and become public charges (Katz 1990; O'Connor 2002). In this book, we use the terms "welfare" and "welfare state" in the more inclusive sense in which Marshall understood it and in the way it is used in discussions of the State's role in the support of citizens in Europe and elsewhere. In this sense, the welfare state consists of all of the social and economic institutions and legislation that provide the material basis for productive citizenship. These institutions and laws include publicly funded education, health care, housing, labor laws, disability insurance, family allowances, public transportation, and more. In the United States, Social Security and Medicare form the core of the middle-class welfare state and they provide nearly universal income support and health care to retirees. To the extent that public parks and hiking trails enhance the quality of life in our highly urbanized world, they too can be considered part of the welfare state (Zuberi 2006). In this sense, middle-class Americans are as much on welfare as are the poor, since few expect to pay for their health care out of pocket or finance their retirements solely from earnings and savings. Middle-class Americans benefit from laws that encourage employers to offer health insurance plans, that insure their retirement plans, and that allow them to save for retirement in tax-deferred investment vehicles.

Along with others we argue that the United States is as much a welfare state as the nations of Europe. Many observers have noted that real social welfare expenditures in the United States are every bit as high as they are in nations with greater public expenditures for social services; they just appear in a different form (Gilbert and Gilbert 1989; Gottschalk 2000; Hacker 2002; Howard 1997; Stevens 1988). In the United States, Medicare and Social Security, tax exempt and deferred retirement and health plans, and other benefits for the middle class account for a major fraction of aggregate expenditures for social welfare. These are paid for out of public funds in the form of foregone tax revenues and represent major direct and indirect investments in citizens' welfare (Hacker 2002).

The fact that a large fraction of total social spending in the United States is indirect and in the form of tax-subsidized benefits for the middle class masks the fact that this form of income distribution represents social welfare expenditure as much as does direct assistance. It improves the lives of individuals by giving them more of what money can buy. Since tax exemptions make people feel that they are simply keeping more of their own money, the public nature of the expense is not as obvious. Yet these middle-class subsidies have a major distributional impact, as well as important implications for the health and welfare of the poor. As Jacob S. Hacker notes, "...it matters fundamentally whether a nation's social welfare framework is characterized by low public spending, low taxes, and high private spending, on the one hand, or high public spending, high taxes, and low private spending, on the other; and this is true even if after-tax spending is identical" (Hacker 2002, p. 23). The immediate consequence of the form of welfare spending characteristic of the United States is a much higher level of inequality and higher rates of poverty than is typical of European welfare states (Smeeding 2000; Smeeding et al. 2001). Clearly, these different social welfare systems and philosophies for providing public goods can result in profound class-based disparities in material well-being.

By the end of the twentieth century, the welfare state was well developed in the rich nations of the world but it faced new and serious challenges. These challenges, which have been made worse by the global economic recession that began in 2008, result from fiscal crises related to the growing cost of providing the full range of social benefits and the realities of a globalized economic system in which individual countries have less control over their internal economies than they did in the period immediately after World War II (Pierson 2001a,b; Swank 2001). Each nation responds to the new international economic reality in its own way, but to varying degrees most countries have experimented with neoliberal reforms and a new "third way" in macroeconomic and labor policies (Campbell 2004; Campbell and Pedersen 2001; Giddens 1998; Romano 2006). This new third way includes attempts to increase economic flexibility and global competitiveness by loosening some of the guarantees that workers fought for and won after Second World War. The essence of these new attempts is to employ market mechanisms to increase productivity, including policies that make it easier to fire workers in economic downturns and to reduce the benefits that have come to define the welfare state.

The almost inevitable retrenchment of welfare states means that the hard-earned social rights of worker and their families are coming under attack (Reich 2007). Since the world's material resources are not infinite, some retrenchment is inevitable, but that fact immediately raises questions about who will pay the greatest cost. For the most part, it is likely to be those who were never all that secure to begin with. Indigenous peoples, immigrants from developing countries, and ethnic minorities figure prominently among these groups. In the United States, African-Americans and Hispanics, along with Native Americans, are among those groups. They benefit from the public expenditures of the welfare state and will suffer the most from cuts, which governments are increasingly forced to impose.

Hispanics and the Retirement Wage

John Myles and others have pointed out that retirement is historically quite a new phenomenon made possible by an adequate "retirement wage," a term that refers to an adequate income that does not depend on work (Myles 1984). Prior to the twentieth century, individuals worked until they were no longer physically able to and then they moved in with children or depended on the charity of others (Bengtson and Achenbaum 1993). Today, employment-based retirement plans and Social Security make it possible for middle-class Americans to retire with some dignity and security. Unfortunately for others, including many Hispanic workers, an adequate retirement wage remains elusive. The fact that their current incomes remain low means that planning for the distant future is pointless. Evidence from survey data indicates that many baby-boom-era Hispanics who will soon reach retirement age have made no retirement plans at all (Lusardi and Mitchell 2007). Low income and the lack of planning have serious negative implications for asset accumulation and for economic well-being in old age (Gassoumis et al. 2008).

Old-Age, Survivors and Disability Insurance (OASDI), or Social Security, is the major public income support program for older Americans. It was designed to protect retirees from severe poverty and it is vital to the large fraction of Hispanic elders who do not have private retirement plans and who are unable to accumulate wealth during their working years (Angel and Angel 1997). Given the universal nature of Social Security, nearly all retired Americans qualify. Yet many older Hispanics, and particularly the foreign-born, do not receive benefits (Fry et al. 2005). Only 76% of Hispanics receive Social Security retirement compared with 91% of non-Hispanic whites and 85% of non-Hispanic blacks (Fry et al. 2005). There are several reasons for nonparticipation by Hispanic workers and nonworkers. Many spent their lives engaged in noncovered employment or they were employed only intermittently or seasonally. Many had multiple Social Security numbers and often their employers failed to make required contributions. When the Social Security program was implemented in 1934, agricultural, seasonal, and domestic workers, occupations with high Hispanic and African-American representation, were not included (Berkowitz 1991). As a consequence, many older minority workers never became part of the program even after those occupations were included (Mintz 2007). Undocumented workers often pay taxes during their working lives but do not collect benefits that they are entitled to later because they fear government reprisal (Smith and Edmonston 1997). Anti-immigrant sentiments that have grown in recent years have had chilling effect that discourages entitled immigrants to ask for services or apply for benefits (de la Garza 2005).

For older Hispanics, then, Social Security is a major component of total income. Forty-four percent of Hispanics in the United States rely on Social Security for at least 90% of their income compared with 29% of non-Hispanic whites (Hendley and Bilimoria 1999). Without Social Security, over half of elderly Hispanics would live in poverty (Torres-Gil et al. 2005). Although Social Security is regressive for the working-age population since only a portion of earnings are taxed, it is progressive in terms of payments since individuals who paid lower taxes because of low earnings receive a higher proportion of their contributions as benefits (Fry et al. 2005). As a consequence, progressive payouts benefit Hispanics who on average have low incomes (National Council of La Raza 2005). Even with this progressive feature, though, without other income, individuals who rely solely on Social Security face a fairly austere economic reality. The average Social Security benefit for all beneficiaries was $9,900 in 2005 but for Hispanics it was only $8,056 (Martin 2007). To strengthen retirement security among Hispanics, then, the National Council of La Raza, a major advocacy and lobbying group for Hispanics, recommends certain improvements to standard retirement plans. These include automatic enrollment in 401(k) plans, increasing the amount of tax-deferred contributions workers can make to IRAs and to 401(k) plans, and eliminating when income and asset tests that are used to determine eligibility for means-tested programs (Orszag and Rodriguez 2005).

This heavy dependence on Social Security will in all likelihood continue (Fry et al. 2005). As a result of an exclusive dependence on a minimal Social Security income, over 600,000 Hispanics aged 65 and over remain in poverty or precariously close to it, and their retirement years are plagued by economic uncertainty (Torres-Gil et al. 2005). A 1997 survey by the Pew Charitable Trusts revealed that approximately one-third of Hispanics who were not currently poor feared that they would descend into poverty in old age. It appears that such fears are based on fact. One study found that while only 5% of working adults in the general population report that they support their parents, more than a third of working Hispanic adults provide financial support to their parents (Metropolitan Life Insurance Company 2005). This financial responsibility for aging parents can undermine a family's ability to save or to educate younger generations. The lack of planning and ability to save for retirement, then, has long-term negative consequences for the Hispanic population generally.

Falling Through the Cracks

As we begin to see, the combination of employment-based benefits system and limited publicly funded social welfare programs in the United States has important implications for minority workers and their families. In the absence of a fully developed welfare state that provides universal health-care coverage and other benefits, those groups that are confined to employment in the service sector, those with episodic and casual employment, and those who are chronically unemployed face potentially serious hardship. To begin to understand the extent of the vulnerability among the Mexican-origin population, we begin with a general overview of retirement plan coverage. In later chapters, we will examine retirement and health-care coverage for men and women of different ages in more detail.

In Figure 1.1, we provide information on the extent of private retirement plan coverage for Hispanics, African-Americans, and non-Hispanic white workers for 2007 from the Survey of Consumer Finances, one of the best sources of information on retirement plan coverage available (Kennickell 2006). Retirement plans include IRA/Keogh accounts and defined-benefit plans. Unfortunately, as is the case with much of data available it is not possible to disaggregate the Hispanic category, but we remind the reader that the largest segment of the Hispanic population consists of individuals of Mexican origin and patterns for the Hispanic group are heavily

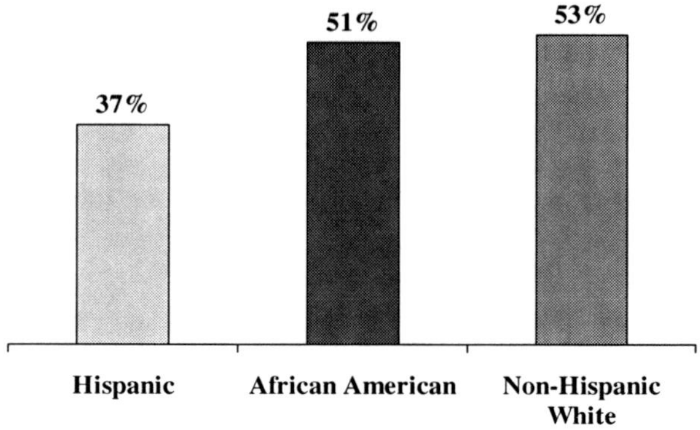

Fig. 1.1 Percentage of individuals 21–64 years with employer-provided retirement plans by race/Hispanic ethnicity (2007)
Source: Survey of Consumer Finances (2007).

influenced by their characteristics. The figure highlights the rather large disparity in private pension coverage among the three groups. Approximately 37% of Hispanics aged 21–64 years had retirement coverage in 2007 compared with over 50% for non-Hispanic whites and African-Americans. These findings are similar to those reported by the National Council of La Raza (2005), one of the leading advocacy groups for the Hispanic population (Orszag and Rodriguez 2005).

Certain evidence suggests that while the difference between African-American and non-Hispanic white workers decreases as income levels increase, a similar convergence does not occur for Hispanics (Copeland 2007). Analyses of the 2007 Current Population Survey (CPS), the major ongoing federal survey that provides information from which such important statistics as the unemployment and poverty rates are computed, show that Hispanics participate at lower rates than other groups at all education levels, including among the college educated (Copeland 2007). Even at higher levels of income Hispanic rates of coverage remain lower than those of other groups. In the CPS while 70% of non-Hispanic whites with incomes of $50,000 or more reported owning a retirement plan, only 57% of Hispanics with incomes in this range reported retirement plans. In addition, as we will demonstrate more fully later, regardless of characteristics such as firm size or job tenure, Hispanics are far less likely to have retirement coverage than non-Hispanic whites or African-Americans.

These low levels of retirement plan participation among Hispanics have serious implications for their retirement security, but what is perhaps even more worrisome is that coverage rates among Hispanics appear to be dropping. While non-Hispanic white participation in employer-sponsored retirement plans increased between 1987 and 2004 from 48% to 52.9%, the Hispanic participation rate decreased during the same period from 32.2% to 28.7% (Copeland 2005). This low rate of coverage results largely from the fact that employers are not required to offer retirement plans to their employees (Schulz and Binstock 2006). Employers who wish to attract highly skilled employees may find that they have no choice but to offer generous benefit packages, but small service sector employers, for whom Hispanic workers are most likely to work, can often simply not afford to. The seriousness of the situation is compounded by the fact that in addition to lacking formal retirement plans, as we noted above, Hispanic workers are less likely than other workers to report that they are saving for retirement (Orszag and Rodriguez 2005).

These low levels of retirement plan participation among Hispanics mask significant within-group differences based on individual and employment characteristics (Greenwald 2007). Native-born Hispanics, for example, are similar to African-Americans in rates of participation, even as both groups' participation is lower than that of non-Hispanic whites (Helman et al. 2007). Foreign-born Hispanics, though, have substantially lower rates of coverage than even African-Americans, regardless of other personal characteristics including age. In addition, Hispanic immigrants are half as likely as native-born Hispanics to have retirement savings or to be currently saving (Helman et al. 2007). It is clear, then, that retirement preparation among Hispanics is inadequate and reflects low levels of human capital. As we will see, low levels of human capital are part of a complex package of disadvantages that make changing the situation of large numbers of Hispanic workers difficult. As an example, one major job characteristic that influences that a worker has a retirement plan is firm size. Small employers operate with low profit margins and are often simply unable to offer benefits. In economic downturns even those that offer retirement plans often must drop them or reduce the employer contribution.

Even though coverage for all workers is lower in small firms than in larger firms, as is the case in so many of the comparisons we present in this and the following chapters, Hispanics fare worse than non-Hispanics even in firms of similar size. Data from the 2007 CPS show that whereas 16% of non-Hispanic white wage and salary workers in firms with fewer than 10 employees participate in a retirement plan, only 7% of Hispanic workers do so (Copeland 2007). Although the level of participation increases for Hispanics in larger firms, the overall disparity in coverage persists in most occupations. Even self-employed Hispanics are less likely than self-employed non-Hispanic white workers with similar levels income to participate in a retirement savings plan or have an IRA (Greenwald 2007).

Even when Hispanics do participate in employer-sponsored 401(k) plans, they contribute less than others. In 2000, the average value of 401(k) plans among households with incomes between $40,000 and $50,000 was $12,136 for Hispanics and $24,909 for non-Hispanics (Orszag and Rodriguez 2005). Given the fact that even among non-Hispanics contributions to 401(k) plans are inadequate to meet retirement needs, this even lower rate of savings among Hispanics is serious. It is possible that part of the problem for such low levels of retirement savings and participation in retirement among Hispanics is a lack of information or knowledge concerning the importance of saving for retirement or the tax-deferred savings opportunities available. This possibility is supported by findings that show Mexican-origin workers, and especially the foreign born, are less likely than non-Hispanic workers to have access to retirement planning services, financial counseling, or advice concerning investing and savings (Orszag and Rodriguez 2005). Less than a quarter of Hispanics have tried to calculate what would be required in terms of savings for a secure retirement (Lusardi and Mitchell 2007). Of course given their low average levels of household income such an exercise may be meaningless. What seems clear though is that as a result of structural disadvantages in the labor force, a large fraction of Mexican-origin families are failing to save for retirement and face an uncertain future.

As the result of low levels of savings and wealth accumulation during their working years and the lack of retirement plans, a large fraction of elderly Mexican-origin individuals find themselves entirely dependent on Social Security or Supplemental Security Income (SSI), the federal program for very poor older Americans. Approximately 13% of Hispanics aged 65 and over receive SSI, compared with 10% of African-American and 3% of non-Hispanic white elders (Social Security Administration 2005). In Chapters 4 and 5, we will return to the issue of retirement security and examine the serious lack of coverage among working-age males and females, and in Chapter 6, we will examine the impact of a lifetime of low savings and the lack of retirement plans on elderly Hispanics. First, though, we turn to health insurance, the second major benefit that guarantees the health and happiness of Americans. As with retirement plans, the employment basis of health insurance coverage in the United States means that because of labor force disadvantages many Hispanic families go without coverage.

Health Insurance Coverage

In addition to a retirement plan, health insurance represents a major employment benefit, one for which unions have negotiated and which defines a good job. As we have noted, health insurance has income support characteristics since in its absence one would have to pay for medical care out of pocket. Hispanic families face both financial and nonfinancial barriers to obtaining health insurance (DeNavas-Walt et al. 2008). These barriers include the same individual and job characteristics, such as low educational levels and employment in firms that do not offer group health insurance coverage, that limit access to employment-based retirement plans. In addition, other factors including low household income, large families, and cultural and linguistic barriers reduce access to health care among Hispanics (Angel et al. 2006). Other barriers include limited access to public insurance due to complicated application and renewal procedures, asset tests, inadequate outreach efforts by agencies charged with administering health-related programs, and eligibility criteria that restrict public program participation only to the poorest families (Angel et al. 2006).

In combination, these barriers result in a serious lack of health-care coverage among Hispanics, and especially among those of Mexican origin. As Figure 1.2, which shows the sources of coverage for working-age adults, reveals Hispanics face particularly serious obstacles to health-care coverage when compared with other groups (Angel and Angel 2007; Santos and Seitz 2000; Treviño et al. 1991). These comparisons are based on a combined sample from the 2004 and 2006 Annual Social and Economic (ASEC) Supplements to the March CPS (U.S. Census

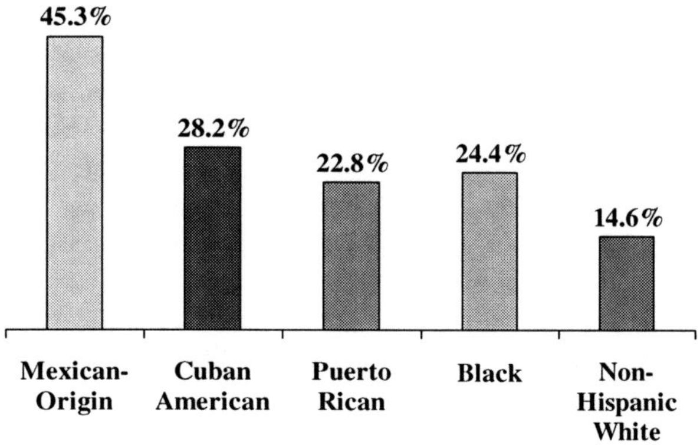

Fig. 1.2 Percentage of individuals 18–64 years without health insurance coverage by race/Mexican-origin ethnicity (2006)
Source: Current Population Survey (2004–2006).

Bureau 2002; 2006a). This combined sample provides a sufficiently large sample of Mexican-origin respondents to allow us to examine them separately. We will use these data throughout the book to examine the situation of the Mexican-origin population and compare it with that of non-Hispanic whites and African-Americans, as well as that of other Hispanic groups. As we will see in many contexts, these data reveal a serious lack of health insurance among Mexican-origin workers. As we will show in subsequent chapters, this serious lack of health insurance coverage begins in infancy and persists throughout the life course for the Mexican-origin population.

As we see, although the majority of working-age non-Hispanic white adults have employer-sponsored health insurance, less than one-half of Mexican Americans participate in employment-based group plans. Approximately one quarter of African-American, Cuban American, and Puerto Rican adults report that they have no health insurance. Yet among those of Mexican origin, nearly half report that they have no health-care coverage of any sort. It is clear from these data and other studies that working-age Mexican-origin individuals are seriously uninsured and underinsured (Schur and Feldman 2000). These statistics underscore the differential vulnerability of various groups. Among Hispanics, factors that are as yet poorly understood affect coverage. These may reflect regional concentration and labor market disadvantages, immigration and citizenship status, language difficulties, and other barriers that increase the risk of inadequate coverage (Schur and Feldman 2000). As stated previously, Mexican Americans are concentrated in low-wage service sector jobs and are far less likely than any other group to be employed in managerial or professional occupations (Fronstin 2005a).

Public Program Participation

It appears, that Hispanics, and particularly those of Mexican origin, are not well served by the private employment-based retirement or health insurance systems that have evolved in the United States. The obvious question that arises, then, is what sources of retirement income and health-care coverage do low-income Hispanics and other poor Americans rely upon? In reality other than private charity the only alternative is the State. Social Security, Medicare, and Medicaid were introduced in order to deal with the most serious areas of need and they have been quite effective in addressing the income and heath-care needs of the elderly and poor children. The glaring omission, though, consists of working-age adults for whom there are few public health-care programs or income supports except for individuals with special medical conditions or those who receive general assistance.

Let us begin by reviewing the role of Social Security in assuring an adequate income for older Hispanics. Social Security is clearly an important income support program, particularly for those who have no private retirement plan. As we show in greater detail in Chapter 6, for about 29% of older Hispanic couples and 45% of single individuals, Social Security is their only source of income (Center for American Progress 2004). Social Security has clearly been a very successful program in terms of income support for the elderly. Since it was introduced in 1935 poverty among the elderly has decreased dramatically (National Bureau of Economic Research 2004). Various aspects of the program make it particularly important for low-wage participants. Although Social Security taxes are regressive during the working years since individuals with high incomes pay only on part of their income (up to $106,800 in 2009), it is progressive in what it pays to recipients (Martin 2007). That means that low-wage workers who contribute less than high-wage workers receive a higher return as a proportion of their contribution than those with higher wages. Older individuals with low incomes also pay lower income taxes than higher income elders.

Social Security was intended to raise low-income older persons out of abject poverty; it was never meant to be a person's sole source of income, and in the absence of a private retirement plan or substantial savings one must live on a relatively modest income. In 2008, a married individual who was 65 years old and making $40,000 a year would have received approximately $19,000 per year in Social Security if he or she had retired. Even with reduced expenditures this is not a great deal of money given what one must pay a Medicare premium and the health expenditures that Medicare does not cover while paying property taxes and other bills. Older individuals who qualify for SSI, the federal program for older adults with very low incomes and few assets, live on even less. In 2008, a couple on SSI received a maximum of $956 a month.

For the working-age population, there is really no means-tested public safety net to compensate for the lack of employment benefits. Income supports, food stamps, housing assistance, Medicaid, and other programs are available for the poorest families, especially those with children or a pregnant female, but relatively few childless adults qualify. In Figure 1.3, we compare participation in Medicaid, SSI, Temporary Aid to Dependent Families (TANF), Food Stamps, child care, and other services among non-Hispanic white, African-American, and Mexican-origin families with family incomes below the official US government poverty level. In 2005, the middle year of the 3 years to which the data refer, the poverty threshold for a family of four with two children was $19,806. A family whose income falls below that level is officially poor and their income to poverty ratio is 1.00 or lower. For the

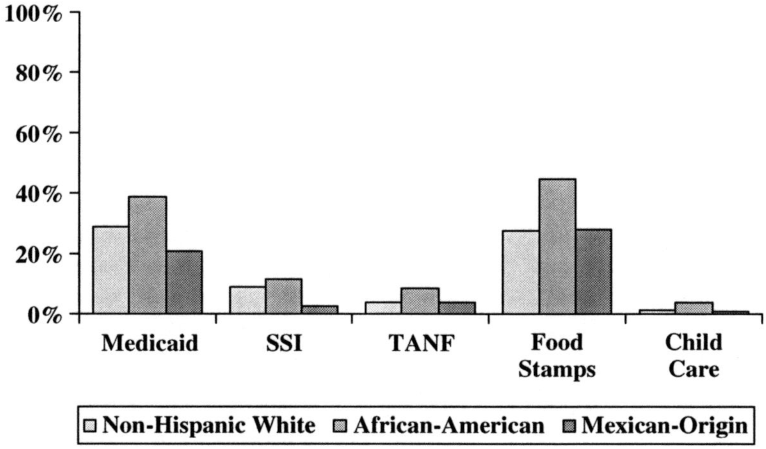

Fig. 1.3 Program participation by families under 100% poverty, 2006
Source: Current Population Survey (2004–2006).

same family of four an income to poverty ratio of 2.00, or twice the poverty level, requires an income of nearly $40,000. The poverty threshold takes the size of the family into account and is regularly adjusted to account for rising prices. Given the fact that means-tested programs are aimed at the poorest families, those with income to poverty ratios of 1.00 or lower, we would expect this group to have the highest participation rates.

If we compare families with incomes this low, we see that Mexican-origin families are less likely than non-Hispanic white or African-American families to participate in Medicaid, SSI, or child care. They are far less likely than African-American families to receive Food Stamps. At higher levels of income relative to poverty, Mexican-origin families continue to participate in Medicaid and SSI at lower rates than the other two groups. In light of low levels of education and the well-documented occupational disadvantages of the Mexican-origin population, this low level of program use in comparison to African-Americans suggests a great deal of unmet need. Children in families with incomes below poverty should almost all qualify for Medicaid or the State Children's Health Insurance Program (SCHIP) (Centers for Medicare and Medicaid Services 2005). The fact that the Mexican-origin population has higher fertility and more children than other groups suggests an even greater problem of underutilization. We begin to find serious evidence that the US welfare state has serious shortcomings for the most needy.

The Long-Term Consequences of Hispanic Exclusion

The point we make is hardly subtle and the data are overwhelming in showing the serious disadvantages that Hispanics, especially those of Mexican origin, experience in terms of retirement and health benefits. Our system of employment-based benefit coverage does not work for poor families, especially those dependent on low-wage jobs, nor does it address the needs of a large fraction of minority Americans. As we document in subsequent chapters, the employment-based benefit deficit among Hispanics has negative consequences for individuals and families from infancy to old age. Low levels of human capital translate directly into low family incomes, and low family incomes taken together add up to low neighborhood and community assets, reducing the group's social and political power. The income disadvantage of minority Americans is fairly well documented but the consequences of the lack of a comprehensive welfare state that insures social rights are not well understood. The fact that the United States does not have a universal health-care financing system has profound implications not only for individual health levels and racial and ethnic disparities in disease burden but also for the nation as a whole.

No one would argue with the statement that avoidable and correctable differences in health and vitality are unfair in and of themselves, but the case for a more comprehensive and equitable health-care system need not be based on considerations of fairness alone. An equitable and comprehensive welfare state that insures everyone's health and provides high-quality education to all citizens is the only way that the United States will maintain its economic superiority in an increasingly globalized world. The reality of our collective social life is that everyone's welfare will at some point depend on the health and productive capacity of others. Our rapidly aging population must be supported by the contributions of those still in the labor force. At the same time, elementary and secondary schools, universities, and public institutions of all sorts depend entirely on the wealth created by those who are currently employed in order to function. The nation's infrastructure is seriously in need of repair and maintenance and again it is the working-age population who must pay for them.

The problem the nation faces is dramatically illustrated by the growing Social Security and Medicare dependency burden. Although some people believe that Social Security acts as a savings plan and that an individual's contributions provide an annuity that generates income for his or her retirement, the system is actually a pay-as-you-go arrangement, a term that is used to refer to the fact that the benefits that retired individuals get come directly from the taxes paid by the working-age population. Therein lies the core problem; in 1945, a decade after Social Security was introduced, there were approximately 40 workers contributing to the support of each retired worker. By 2003 that number had shrunk to slightly more than three, and by 2030 only two workers will contribute to the support of each retire (Social Security Administration 2004). If the program remains a pay-as-you-go system in which the support of the retired population comes directly from the paychecks of those who are still working, each employed American will have to contribute a huge, and probably prohibitive, fraction of his or her income to Social Security and Medicare for the elderly (Bongaarts 2004). In addition to supporting the retired population, the future labor force will be called upon to pay for defense and our other national priorities.

The looming problem of the support of a growing retired population is made more serious by the fact that the high growth rates and the relative youth of the

Hispanic populations will make up an ever-growing fraction of the future labor force. If the educational levels of these Hispanic workers remain low and if their productivity is compromised by poor health, the productive potential of the economy as a whole will be placed in serious jeopardy. In the absence of a comprehensive welfare state that insures high-quality education, health care, safe housing, and adequate income, the productive potential of the future labor force seems doomed to decrease at a time when the economic burden on it will increase.

The economic crisis of 2008, which at this writing is the worst economic downturn in decades, makes the need for an economic stimulus package clear. Among the items that have been discussed as central items in a stimulus package is education, especially for low-income children. The crisis makes the short-term need for job creation clear but it also draws our attention to the longer term needs of the American labor force. For years educators and social critics have been aware of the fact that America's economic productive potential depends on an educated labor force. In order to compete with China, India, and other emerging economies, American workers must become ever more productive. That means that Hispanic workers must become ever more productive since they will make up a growing fraction of the total labor force. Without serious investment in the health and welfare of Hispanic families and youth, the productive potential of the American labor force will be forfeited and the United States of the future will be relegated to the position of one of the less economically powerful nations. A comprehensive welfare state is more than the dream of a few social progressives; it represents the only real hope for the future. Despite concerns over the cost of universal programs such as universal health care, balancing budgets by shortchanging those programs that would guarantee the future is simply eating the seed corn. It represents a short-term solution to a short-term problem but with potentially devastating long-term consequences.

In the chapters that follow, we will reveal the conditions in which a large segment of the future labor force is spending its childhood and adolescence. These conditions are not conducive to the development of the highest levels of physical, emotional, or social health. As we will show, the health and economic risks that these future workers face are the result of structural factors related to the labor market in which their parents find employment and the incomplete nature of the social welfare safety net that guarantees their health and welfare. Those children who today suffer serious educational and other disadvantages, and who will as a consequence find themselves restricted to low-wage occupations in adulthood, will not have the resources nor will they likely be willing to shoulder the burden of supporting a disproportionately non-Hispanic white elderly population (Angel and Angel 2006). This racial and ethnic overlay lends a potentially explosive dimension to the crisis of the support of an aging retired population at the same time that our nation will face new challenges in the war on terror, the education of the young, the decay of our metropolitan areas, and serious global economic competition.

Chapter 2
The Latin Americanization of the US Labor Force

Unlike the nations of Europe that have only recently begun to accept the fact that they are nations of immigrants, the United States has been defined by immigration throughout its history. In the eighteenth and nineteenth centuries, immigrants from the nations of Europe contributed to the great diversity in national and cultural origins that define the nation. At the turn of the century, most Americans lived in small towns and on farms (Portes and Rumbaut 2006), but a dynamic economy and growing urban centers provided new immigrants ample opportunity for employment in construction and manufacturing and a chance to move up the economic ladder. After two or three generations, the children of these immigrants became fully assimilated middle-class Americans. The common assumption that informed classic theoretical models of incorporation and assimilation was that over time the cacophony of languages and cultures that defined immigrant America would give way to English and a common American cultural identity. Although such a blending of different ethnic groups has indeed occurred, at least for Americans of European origin, the continual infusion of new cultures and languages means that the United States today is as diverse as it ever was. What is different today, though, is the fact that the new immigrants are no longer from Europe. For the last few decades, the vast majority of immigrants have come from Asia and Latin America (He 2002), a fact that has significant implications for the racial and ethnic composition of the future labor force.

Traditionally, Hispanics have been geographically concentrated. Those of Mexican origin remained in the southwestern United States, which until the end of the nineteenth century was part of Mexico. Puerto Ricans and Dominicans have historically settled in the cities of the northeast, and Cubans fled their home island to recreate Little Havana in Florida. Today, Spanish language television and radio can be heard in the heartland and in southeastern states in places that until recently had never known Hispanics. Although the majority of Americans are still white and non-Hispanic, by the middle of the twenty-first century approximately one-half of all Americans will trace their heritage to Africa, Asia, or Latin America (Passel and Cohn 2008). Individuals from Latin America and Asia are redefining the cultural landscape of California and Texas and becoming important economic and political forces in other states as well (Hayes-Bautista 2004). Despite the anti-immigrant sentiment that informs much public discussion related to the Hispanic population, the

R.J. Angel, J.L. Angel, *Hispanic Families at Risk*, DOI 10.1007/978-1-4419-0474-4_2,

labor needs of the nation will in all likelihood continue to attract both legal and illegal immigrants. Immigration and high fertility mean that the Hispanic population is relatively young and will make up a growing fraction of the population and the labor force in the years to come (U.S. Census Bureau, 2009). Today, one-third of Hispanics, but only a quarter of non-Hispanics, are under the age of 18 years (Tienda and Mitchell 2006b). In the future, the levels of productivity of the Hispanic population will affect the nation's overall level of material welfare and global power.

Although most Hispanics are native born, immigration is a central demographic and cultural phenomenon for the population as a whole. In this chapter, we draw upon the group's immigrant experience to explain the marginalized status of segments of the Hispanic population. Even after several generations in this country, many Hispanics remain trapped in the lower class. For them, the immigration experience has not led to the American dream. Theirs is a story of failed incorporation into the economic and political mainstreams. In this and subsequent chapters, we examine the consequences of that failed incorporation for the population's access to the social rights we elaborated in the first chapter and delve into its possible causes. The extent of the problem is massive and made ever more serious by the serious economic downturn that began in 2008. Even for the Mexican-origin population of the Southwest who were basically colonized when the northern part of Mexico was annexed in 1848 after the Mexican war, the outsider metaphor still holds. Issues of cultural and racial difference, then, are central to the story of Hispanic incorporation and the issue of coexistence and economic success must be understood in the context of significant differences from the mainstream.

Multiculturalism and Diversity

Richard Alba, a keen observer of American ethnicity, observed some years ago that since the large-scale European immigration that created the ethnic diversity of nineteenth century urban America ended long ago, distinctions between Americans of European origin have all but disappeared. Today, differences between individuals of English, German, French, and other nationalities have been replaced by a common American cultural identity (Alba 1990). There can be little doubt that distinctions among Americans of European origin are less obvious or socially significant than those between European-origin Americans as a whole and African-Americans, Asians, and Latinos. In addition to representing minority groups, Americans of Asian and Latin American origin differ significantly among themselves. Latinos with roots in the Caribbean are very different from those who emigrated from Mexico or those who have lived in the American Southwest since it was part of Mexico. Puerto Ricans are full US citizens whether they were born on the mainland or on the island of Puerto Rico, Cuban-Americans are political refugees, and Mexicans are for the most part economic migrants.

Unlike Asians, Hispanics at least share a common core language, Spanish. In addition to variation in their nations of origin, differences among Latinos arise from the fact that the different nationalities arrived at different historical moments and settled in different parts of the country, factors that have influenced their social and occupational opportunities (Montes de Oca, Molina, and Avalos 2008; Portes and Bach 1985; Portes and Rumbaut 1996, 2006). California is home to both old-time Hispanic families that have been in the state for generations and more recent immigrants. Other cities and states have seen rapid recent growth in their Hispanic populations, and especially the Mexican-origin population (Suro and Singer 2002). Los Angeles, with over 1 million residents of Mexican origin, has the largest Mexican-origin population in the country; Chicago, with over one-half million Mexican-origin residents, is second largest (U.S. Census Bureau 2003).

The growth in the Mexican-origin population is fueled both by high fertility and by immigration from Mexico. High rates of immigration and especially the presence of a large number of undocumented immigrants cause great concern among Americans based on fears concerning security, cultural identity, and the potential that new immigrants will become public charges. Problems related to the control of borders and the incorporation of immigrants are not solely concerns in the United States. Most developed nations of the world are facing a new reality of cultural diversity. The massive international migration of peoples from the poor nations of the South to the developed nations of the North represents a core component of the process of globalization that is fundamentally redefining the nation state system and that makes it clear that labor and capital are increasingly international commodities (Balibar 2004; Lucas 2008). This new economic and demographic reality is driven by the lack of opportunities in developing nations and the need for cheap labor in the developed nations. Despite the economic need for immigrant labor, the new immigrants are feared because of their racial, cultural, and religious differences and almost everywhere face strong opposition.

The fear of immigrants, which often accompanies a fear of minority group members and indigenous peoples as well, is driven by deeply held prejudices concerning security and cultural identity. Strident demands for secure borders in the United States, Europe, and elsewhere, and the rise of anti-immigrant sentiments form central planks in the political platforms of political parties of the far right (Huntington 2004), but they are not confined to xenophobic extremists. The real or perceived threats to national solidarity and identity force even centrist parties to take stronger stances toward immigration, and especially illegal immigration. The result is that the demographic and economic reality of developed nations results in fundamental conflicts between restrictive immigration policies and the needs of competitive labor markets (Casteles 2004; Flynn 2005). Few countries do all that might be possible to seal borders and discourage undocumented immigration.

Because of high levels of immigration, modern cities are as racially and ethnically heterogeneous as ever, if in fact they are not more so. Like the United States, the European Union, Australia, Canada, and other developed nations confront a new multiethnic reality that accompanies a highly dynamic global economy with relatively inexpensive forms of long-distance transportation. Given the low fertility of much of Europe, in as little as one generation, the cultural homogeneity that many Europeans remember will be a thing of the past. Tomorrow's Western Europe will be a mosaic of Eastern Europeans, Latin Americans, Africans, and Asians with a generous overlay of Islam. The need for groups that differ in race, ethnicity, cultural practices, and religion introduces serious challenges to attempts to create truly multicultural and inclusive societies.

This new reality forces us to reexamine traditional theories of immigrant incorporation. Certain assimilation models, those of both early and more recent observers, view the United States as a melting pot in which immigrant groups undergo a process of assimilation and acculturation until they no longer view themselves nor are they viewed by others as outsiders (Alba and Nee 2003; Gans 1992; Gordon 1964; Perlmann and Waldinger 1997). This relatively rapid, if not always smooth, process might characterize the experience of the white European immigrants of the nineteenth and early twentieth centuries, but it does not accurately describe the situation of African Americans who arrived in this country as slaves, nor does it necessarily reflect the experiences of more recent immigrants from Latin America (Portes and Rumbaut 2001). It also does not accurately characterize the experience of the longer term Mexican-origin residents of the Southwest who became citizens when a large part of Mexico was annexed to the United States. For Hispanics, and especially those of Mexican origin, the economic and social incorporation process has been more differentiated, or as it has come to be referred to, it has been a more segmented process. As we discussed earlier, the term "segmented" refers to the fact that although a large fraction of Hispanic immigrants have successfully ascended into the middle class and become acculturated, a substantial segment remains permanently trapped in the lower social classes, often taking on the economic and social characteristics of an underclass (Portes et al. 2005; Portes and Zhou 1993; Telles and Ortiz 2008).

Incorporation or Permanent Marginality?

This new immigrant and minority group reality undermines the myth of rapid or easy economic incorporation. Unlike earlier European immigrants to the United States from Europe who were white and Christian or Jewish, recent immigrants to Europe, the United States, and other nations are often racially and culturally very different than the host groups. This fact can create serious barriers to full incorporation, especially if the new arrivals do not wish to shed their culture and assimilate completely, or if they see no incentive to do so. The same is actually true for many longer term minority group residents. Those observers who believe that full cultural assimilation is necessary for social cohesion see serious dangers in the retention or excess affirmation of ethnic or racial group identities. They fear that such specific identities can undermine or prevent the evolution of a common national identity and a sense of common purpose (Schlesinger 1992). Unfortunately, not all groups are granted the opportunity of full economic incorporation or cultural assimilation. In many nations marginalized groups, including indigenous peoples, racially and culturally distinct immigrants, religious minorities, and others are denied the opportunity to fully assimilate even if they wish to; often they do not. Rather than abandon all aspects of their cultures of origin, they would prefer to maintain aspects of that culture.

The adjective "multicultural" and the noun "multiculturalism" have been adopted to refer to an idealized situation in which cultural and religious differences are recognized as legitimate and respected by different groups (Fraser and Honneth 2003; Kymlicka 1995, 2007; Kymlicka and Norman 2000; Taylor 1994). We might ask how these concerns apply to Hispanics and whether they retain the option of continuing to speak Spanish and identify with their cultures of origin, or whether in order to succeed they must abandon those cultural markers. In a truly multicultural society, culturally distinct groups would be free to speak their native languages, practice their religions, and live their private lives in accordance with their own cultural beliefs and practices while participating fully in the larger economic and political institutions.

Unfortunately for many groups such as the Turks in Germany or North Africans in France, neither assimilation nor multicultural acceptance seems likely. Rather than dignity and respect, the reality they face includes cultural and racial stigma coupled with economic and social exclusion. These new immigrants, much like older excluded minority groups, often find that rather than enjoying the rights of citizens, or denizens who share many rights of citizens and who can look forward to the possibility of eventually becoming citizens, they face the reality of permanent residential and social marginalization (Lewis 2005; Lewis and Neal 2005). The fact that the new immigrants are racially, ethnically, and culturally different than the receiving populations gives this segregation a distinctly racist aspect (Schierup et al. 2006). In many cases, assimilation is not a choice since exclusion based on group membership can be imposed by the way a society is structured.

Characteristics of the Hispanic Population

In the remainder of the chapter, we characterize the Hispanic population and summarize the social and economic forces that are affecting its size, distribution, and its relatively low levels of social mobility. We pay particular attention to education since the educational levels of segments of this population, especially for those of Mexican origin who make up the majority of the Hispanic population, remain extremely low (Telles and Ortiz 2008). These low levels of education seriously undermine possibilities for upward mobility for individuals, but they also reduce the level of social capital for the group as a whole (Borjas 1985). Until a substantial number of Hispanics enter the professions and academia, young Hispanics will lack the role models they need to inculcate the middle-class values related to higher levels of education that lead to upward mobility (Kùna and Prieto 2009). Until Hispanic subgroups have a critical mass of articulate analysts and advocates who can frame issues of exclusion and powerlessness effectively in the mainstream media, the voice of the group as a whole will remain unheard. As we argue throughout this book, low educational levels keep the population from gaining access to the highest corridors of power and from achieving adequate representation in the professions and the academy. Without an educated and articulate group of individuals who can frame the question of exclusion and further the core agenda of the group as a whole, little progress will be made toward equity. In the last chapter, we cite the feminist movement's success in framing issues related to gender exclusion as an effective example of what is necessary.

We begin by documenting the rapid growth of the Hispanic population and draw upon a portrait of the Hispanic population provided by the Pew Hispanic Center that includes detailed analyses of the Mexican-origin population. This portrait is based on Census data for 2000 and on data from the American Community Survey for 2006 (Pew Hispanic Center 2008). In 2000, Hispanics accounted for 12.5% of the population of the United States, but by 2006 they made up 14.8%. During those 6 years, the proportion of non-Hispanic whites dropped from 69.1 to 66.2%, while the African-American share of the population remained basically constant at ~12%. The Mexican-origin population makes up the vast majority of Hispanics, 64%, and a large fraction were born in Mexico. In 2007, nearly 40% of the approximately 30 million Mexican-origin individuals in the United States were foreign-born. This large foreign-born representation gives the group unique characteristics. The foreign-born cling to more traditional values and they are more likely to be married. In 2007 while only about 43% of native-born Mexican-origin women over the age of 18 years had ever been married, over 61% of foreign-born women had been married (original analysis from the Current Population Survey).

In addition to high levels of immigration, the growth in the Hispanic population is fueled by high fertility. In 2007, nearly 22% of births in the United States were to Hispanics, with nearly 12% to foreign-born women. Mexican-origin births accounted for over 15% of all births in 2007, with births to foreign-born Mexican-origin women accounting for nearly 9% of the total number of births in the nation. Together, then, immigration and high fertility represent a demographic engine that will maintain the growth rate of the Hispanic and Mexican-origin populations for some time (Ramirez 2004). As we emphasize throughout this book, this growth in the Hispanic population, as well as the age distribution that results, has particularly important implications for the ethnic composition of the future labor force. Figure 2.1, which is based on 2000 Census data, dramatically illustrates the extent of ethnic-age grading of the population of Texas, a state that has a large Mexican-origin population. The figure shows that in 2000, 44% of infants under the age of 5 years were of Mexican-origin, whereas only 40% were non-Hispanic white. At the other end of the age range, only about 17% of Texans over the age of 65 years were of Mexican origin, whereas nearly 73% were non-Hispanic white.

Texas, California and the other states of the Southwest have large Mexican-origin populations, but the phenomenon of growing younger minority populations is not confined to any one region (U.S. Census Bureau 2003). Mississippi, Tennessee, North Carolina, and other states have experienced rapid growth in their Hispanic populations as these groups seek economic opportunities in new areas and take jobs for which no other workers are available (Suro and Singer 2002). The implications for the composition of the future labor force are obvious. By the year 2040, well over half of the Texas labor force will be Hispanic (Murdock et al. 2002). Although Texas may represent an extreme case because of the size of the state's Mexican-origin population, in most of the rest of the country the working-age population will

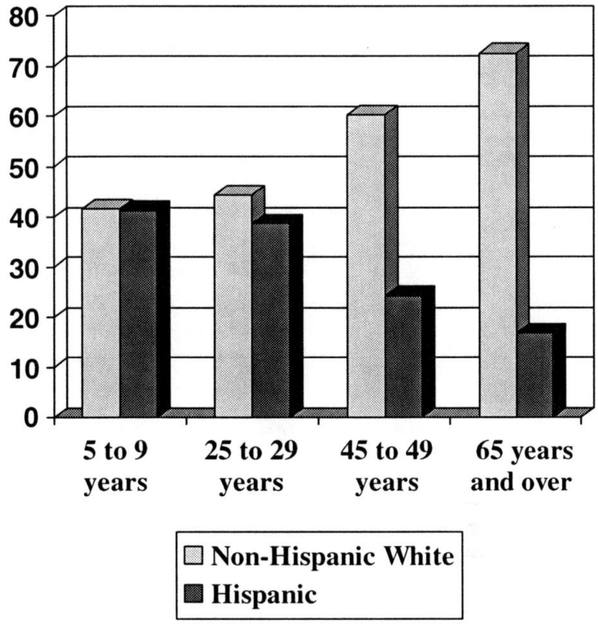

Fig. 2.1 Percent of Texas population by age group and ethnicity, 2000
Source: Murdock, S. H. 2004. *Population change in Texas: Implications for human and socioeconomic resources in the 21st century, slide #30.* San Antonio, TX: The University of Texas at San Antonio.

be disproportionately minority in the relative short-term. This fact has profound implications for social stability and the pact between the generations.

Figure 2.2 lists the 10 metropolitan areas with the highest Hispanic growth rates in the nation between 1990 and 2000. The increase in the Hispanic populations of the southern cities on the list is truly remarkable. In the Charlotte-Concord, South Carolina metropolitan area, for example, the Hispanic population grew by over 600% in just 10 years. The population of Raleigh, North Carolina, grew by over 500%. Outside of the South, Portland, Las Vegas, and Indianapolis experienced large increases in their Hispanic populations. More recent data from the Census bureau indicate that the growth rates of the Hispanic population outside of its traditional locations are continuing and parts of the country that at one time had no Hispanics are rapidly becoming heavily Latino. In 1990 approximately 85% of Mexican immigrants settled in California, Texas, and Illinois, but by 2000 that proportion had declined to 68% as the result of the more diverse set of destinations (The American Immigration Law Foundation 2002).

In the future then, Hispanics will constitute a larger proportion of the population at large and of the labor force in particular. As a result, the economy of the United States will increasingly depend on the productivity of a heavily Hispanic labor force. The collective economic welfare of the nation will therefore depend on their productivity. In 1945 there were 41.9 workers for every retired person receiving Social Security; by 2030 each retiree will depend on the contributions of slightly more than two workers (Social Security Administration 2004b). If a large fraction of those workers are confined to the low-paying service sector they will simply not be able to bear the burden. The impending retirement of the baby-boom generations requires

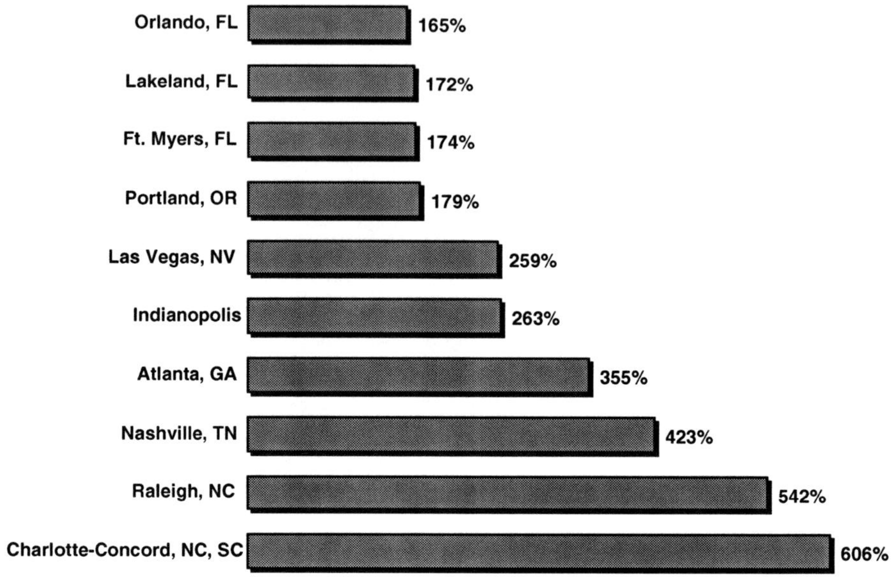

Fig. 2.2 Ten metro areas with highest Hispanic growth rates, 1990–2000
Source: Frey (2006).

huge investments in the education of those who will support them. Unfortunately, as we document throughout the book, that is not happening and the consequences are potentially serious. The United States faces the real possibility of rapid and extensive economic decline. In addition, the ethnic-age grading of the population of the future introduces an ethnic dimension to our system of social stratification that could have serious political consequences. The fact that the productive potential of a large segment of the future labor force might be undermined by poor health and low educational levels has profound implications for older as well as younger Americans. Everyone's welfare depends on the productivity of minority Americans. Yet, as we demonstrate next, the data related to education present a disturbing picture.

Low educational levels among Hispanics represent a major structural weakness in the economy of the United States. Let us review data that illustrate the magnitude of the problem. Figure 2.3 provides information on high school graduation rates for non-Hispanic whites, African-Americans, and three Hispanic subgroups for 2007 from the US Department of Education. These data clearly reveal the disastrous situation in the Mexican-origin population. While 94% of non-Hispanic whites and 88% of African-Americans have graduated from high school, only 65% of Mexican-origin adults have graduated. This is a rate that is substantially lower than those of Puerto Ricans or Cubans and reveals the uniquely serious problem for Mexican-origin adults. There are other aspects of this educational deficit that bode ill for the future of the labor force.

Figure 2.4 presents the data on high school graduation rates separately by gender for non-Hispanic whites, African-Americans, and the combined Hispanic category.

Fig. 2.3 High school graduation rate by race and Hispanic nationality (25–29 years old), 2007
Source: National Center for Education Statistics (2007a).

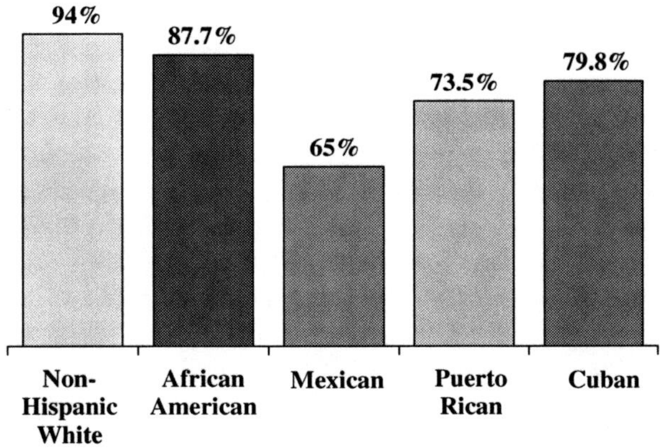

Fig. 2.4 High school graduation rate by gender, race, and Hispanic ethnicity (25 years and over), 2007
Source: National Center for Education Statistics (2007a).

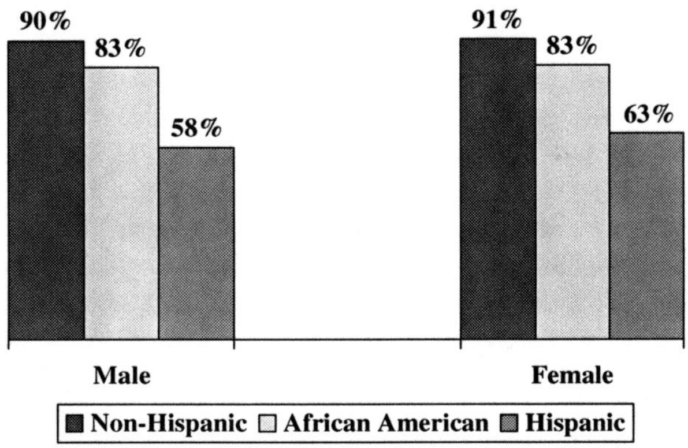

It shows that among Hispanics males have lower graduation rates than females. In addition to all of the other negative consequences associated with low levels of education, they may eventually undermine family life. Currently, Hispanics are more likely to be married and have intact families than non-Hispanics. However, with such low levels of education Hispanic males may find themselves increasingly unable to provide for their families and Hispanic females may find themselves in a very different marriage market with fewer marriageable males. Such a situation limits the potential source of mates for African-American females (Catanzarite and Ortiz 2002). For Hispanics in general, and for the Mexican-origin population in particular, low rates of high school completion bode ill for the future. Without a high school degree, higher levels of educational attainment are not possible and individuals with such low levels of education are at elevated risk of crime and a life of disorganization and poverty. The large numbers of such poorly educated individuals means that a huge potential in terms of human capital will never be realized. The situation is particularly dire in states like California, Illinois, and Texas, which have large Mexican-origin populations.

Let us delve further into the problem of low educational attainment among Hispanics in order to understand other important aspects of the educational deficit.

As we mentioned earlier, the vast majority of Hispanic men are economically active. Hispanic students 16–24 years of age accounted for about 40% of high school dropouts in 2005 (Child Trends 2005). The situation is even worse for the foreign born, fewer than half of whom graduate from high school (Lowell and Suro 2002). Although the situation has improved recently among younger immigrants, high school graduation rates are particularly low among the older immigrant population (Lowell and Suro 2002; Wojtkiewicz and Donato 1995). Among Hispanics, those of Mexican origin have the lowest level of educational attainment. In 2000, only 46% of the Mexican-origin population aged 25 years and older had received at least a high school diploma (Ramirez 2004). Unless the educational level of this population increases dramatically and rapidly, the working-age population of the future will be characterized by low productivity and low income. These lower educational levels and the large number of recent immigrants among Hispanics translate into lower household incomes for young working-age families (Angel and Angel 2006). Almost one-quarter of Hispanic immigrant households reported annual household incomes of less than $20,000 in 2006, while 17% of non-Hispanic whites report incomes that low (Pew Hispanic Center 2006).

The low high school graduation rate is one clear indicator of the seriousness of the educational deficit among Hispanics, but there are other aspects of the educational experience to consider, including the nature and content of the courses that students take. As Fig. 2.5 reveals, among high school students, Hispanics are less likely than non-Hispanic whites or African-Americans to pursue a college preparatory curriculum and they are less likely to take coursework in math and science. Even when they do complete high school, Hispanics are not as prepared as non-Hispanics to major in subjects in college that require a strong mathematical background. Not only do the physical sciences require a strong background in mathematics, but the social sciences do as well as the amount of quantitative data available for social research and planning explodes. Increasingly, leadership positions in business, government, and the academy require advanced degrees and a proven ability to analyze complex data and explain it clearly.

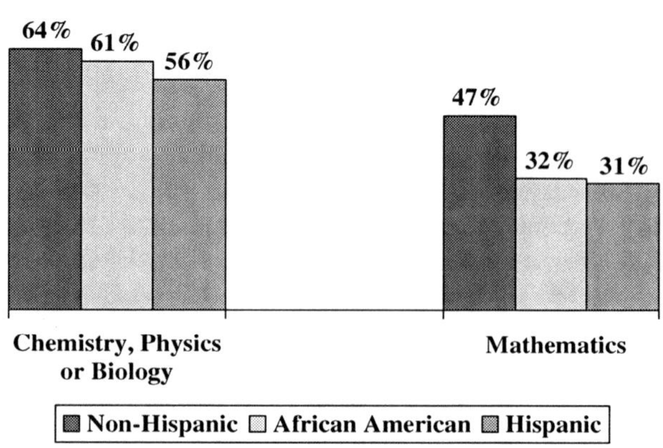

Fig. 2.5 High school graduates who completed advanced science and mathematics courses by race and Hispanic ethnicity, 2000 *Source:* National Center for Education Statistics (2004).

Pathways to Higher Education

The fact that large numbers of minority youth do not graduate from high school or are poorly prepared for college work even when they do limits their future educational possibilities. One indicator of the more limited higher education options is revealed by the fact that even when they go on to post-secondary education, Hispanics are more likely than non-Hispanic whites and African-Americans to attend a 2-year college rather than enroll in a 4-year institution. Of the 1.7 million Hispanic students pursuing post-secondary education, approximately 640,000, or 38.3%, attend 2-year institutions (Kohler and Lazarin 2007). Only 28.3% of non-Hispanic white and 28.1% of African-American students pursuing a post-secondary education are enrolled in 2-year colleges. Figure 2.6 presents comparisons of the proportion of all higher education degrees that are from 2-year colleges by race and Hispanic ethnicity. It shows that for non-Hispanic white males 23% of all degrees are from 2-year institutions, while among Hispanic males 35% of all post-secondary degrees are from 2-year institutions. While graduation from a 2-year program can prepare one for a good job in many areas, 2-year degrees do not qualify one for the highest administrative or professional positions. Clearly some students transfer from a 2-year to a 4-year college, but many do not. In fact only one out of five community college students eventually earns a bachelor's degree (Long and Kurlaender 2008).

Fig. 2.6 Two-year degrees conferred by gender, race, and Hispanic as a percentage of all post-secondary degrees, 2003–2004
Source: National Center for Education Statistics (2005).

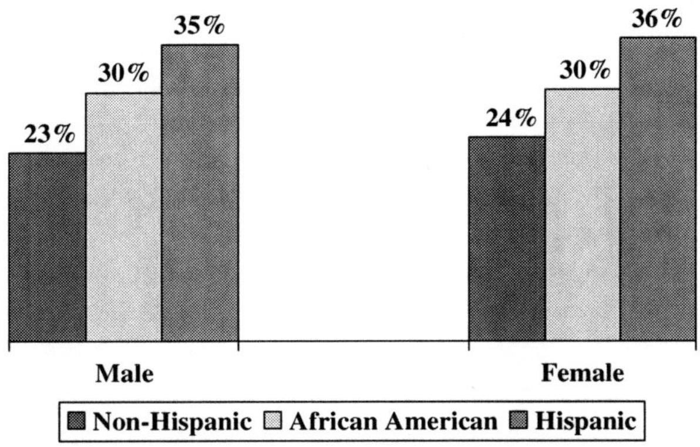

Lower rates of enrollment in 4-year colleges and lower graduation rates represent a further barrier to the accumulation of material and social capital for the Hispanic population. While the proportion of Hispanics who graduate from 4-year institutions of higher learning has nearly doubled since 1960, they are far less likely than non-Hispanic whites and blacks to receive a diploma (National Center for Education Statistics 2007c). Figure 2.7 shows that in 2007, 12% of Hispanic males and 14% of Hispanic females had received a baccalaureate degree compared with 18% of African-American males and 19% of African-American females. College education among non-Hispanic white males is nearly three times higher than that of Hispanic males. Non-Hispanic white females are over twice as likely to have at least a bachelor's degree than Hispanic females (National Center for Education Statistics 2007c).

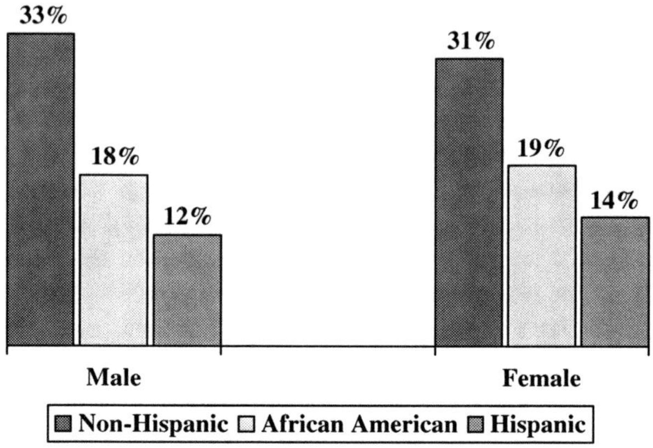

Fig. 2.7 College graduation rate by gender, race, and Hispanic ethnicity, 2007 *Source:* National Center for Education Statistics (2007b).

Figure 2.8 again shows the unique problem of low educational levels among Mexican-origin adults. This figure presents the proportion of non-Hispanic white, African-American, and three Hispanic group adults aged 25–29 years who have earned a bachelor's degree or higher. Only 8% of Mexican-origin young adults have a bachelor's or advanced degree. This is far lower than non-Hispanic whites, but also substantially lower than African-Americans or the other two Hispanic groups. The reasons for this astonishingly low level of higher education are no doubt complex and probably include such factors as a student's preparation in high school, his or her self-concept and educational ambition, family support, peer influences, parental expectations, financial resources, and institutional factors (Pino 2005). What seems clear is that this confluence of factors has a devastating effect on college graduation rates. The result is a population in which children and adolescents do not expect most adults to have high levels of education and commensurate occupational ambitions. As we argue throughout the book, until there is a sufficiently large group of Hispanics, and especially much larger groups of Mexican-origin men and women

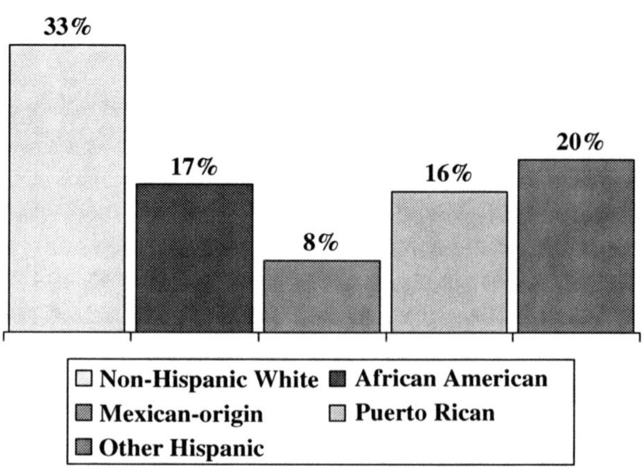

Fig. 2.8 Individuals 25–29 years old with a bachelor's degree or higher by race and Hispanic nationality, 2005 *Source:* National Center for Education Statistics (2007b).

with a college education or more, large segments of this population will remain trapped in the lower social classes.

Clearly it is imperative to attempt to keep adolescents in school and to improve their performance while they are there. Educators and advocates for the Hispanic and Mexican-origin population have worked for years to improve primary and secondary educational outcomes (The Association for the Advancement of Mexican Americans 2009). Bilingual educational programs as well as other interventions have been tried with only limited success (Crosnoe 2006). Such efforts are necessary and laudable but often focus on those with little chance of succeeding educationally. While some may consider it as elitist to focus on the segment of Hispanic students with the greatest educational potential in an attempt to increase their chances of success in higher education, unless more Hispanic students go on to become doctors, lawyers, and other professionals the population as a whole will lack economic and political power. At the same time that we do whatever is necessary to keep students in high school through graduation, it is imperative as well to make sure that those with the intellectual and social resources to succeed have the chance to obtain the highest quality post-secondary educations at the nation's leading institutions of higher learning.

As complex as the predictors of the lack of college and university educations among Hispanics may be, the lack of funding is certainly a critical determinant. The amount of funding available clearly influences a student's decision as to whether and where to attend college, what to major in, and where to live (Pino 2005). A good student from a middle-class family can often pay for his or her education with parental contributions and scholarships and graduate debt-free. For many students, and especially those whose families have limited resources, loans and other forms of financial aid are necessary. In general, Hispanic students receive less financial aid than non-Hispanic white or African-American students (Kohler and Lazarin 2007). The lack of access to financing is probably one of the major reasons as to why many Hispanic students do not finish college or delay graduation. It also affects the probability of continuing on to graduate or professional school. Figure 2.9 shows that Hispanics are greatly underrepresented in graduate and professional schools.

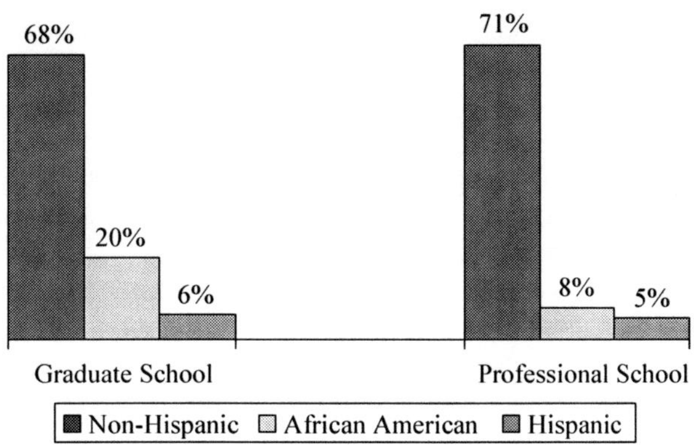

Fig. 2.9 Graduate and professional school enrollment by gender, race, and Hispanic ethnicity
Source: National Center for Education Statistics (2007c).

While nearly 15% of the population at large is Hispanic, only 6% of those attending graduate school and 5% of those attending professional schools are Hispanic.

Educational Barriers to the Professions

These statistics show that the educational deficits among Hispanics, and especially among those of Mexican origin, are serious and it is clear that they will be difficult to correct. Unfortunately, Hispanics and other minority Americans have not been as successful in reversing historical disadvantages as one might have hoped. Although feminists have been able to frame the problem of gender inequality in various areas of life as a structural problem that requires direct solutions, minority Americans have not been as successful in framing the inequities that affect them as the result of historically determined structural factors that must be directly addressed. Calls for the direct redress of previous disadvantages are greeted as examples of special group privilege or reverse discrimination. In the absence of programs that guarantee admission to higher education to representative numbers of Hispanics and other minority students, coupled with targeted programs to make up for inadequate secondary educations, the chances for upward mobility for the group as a whole will remain limited.

It is true that traditional programs aimed at reducing high school dropout rates and supporting minority students in college are insufficient to greatly increase the number of highly educated Hispanic professionals. The traditional liberal approach to the problem of low educational achievement is to focus on elementary and secondary education where the foundation for future success rests. However, as we have said before, in the absence of a significant number of Hispanics with advanced degrees, such efforts will probably continue to see limited success. In our opinion it is imperative to get as many students as possible through college and into graduate and professional schools in the short run. The level of financial support is critical to educational success and includes funding for student support services, student mentoring, one-on-one career counseling, informational programs concerning graduate education, and a substantial increase in the number of Hispanic faculty.

In addition to increased institutional commitment, enhancing the networks outside the university environment is very important in the development of knowledge of and positive expectations concerning possible career pathways. Because the Hispanic family plays such an important role in the lives of its children, it is necessary to change parental expectations concerning their children's education. Numerous observers have noted the desire among Mexican-origin parents that their children remain close to home, which means that they often cannot take advantage of the best educational opportunities. Again, an increased number of highly educated role models can communicate to the Hispanic community the necessity of a broader perspective and the realization that social mobility often means abandoning traditional practices and familiar environments.

Low levels of college, graduate school, and professional school graduation mean that the pool of Hispanic faculty, and especially Mexican-origin faculty, at colleges and universities remains small. According to the National Center for Education Statistics (2006), about 15% of US faculty in colleges and universities were minorities in 2003. Approximately 6% of faculty members were African-American and less than 4% were Hispanic. Nearly half of college faculty members (47%) were non-Hispanic white males and 36% were non-Hispanic white females. Minority representation at the nation's elite research and teaching institutions remains extremely low even in states with large Hispanic populations. At the University of Texas at Austin, the authors' home institution, located in a state in which over 35% of the population is Hispanic, 81.6% of faculty members are non-Hispanic white, 3.7% are African-American, and only 5.8% are Hispanic (U.T. Office of Information and Management 2007).

The Core Barrier to Group Mobility

We end this chapter by reiterating the profound negative impact of low levels of education on Hispanic occupational job opportunities, income, and wealth. The mechanism by which low levels of education affect income and wealth is, of course, through occupation. Professional occupations which pay well and allow one to save and accumulate wealth require high levels of education. Individuals with low levels of education are confined to low-wage jobs in agriculture, construction, and the service sector. Figure 2.10 shows the proportion of Hispanic workers in major occupational categories. The data are quite telling and show that only 6.8% of professionals are Hispanic, whereas 39.7% of agricultural workers are Hispanic. Relative to their population representation, Hispanics are overrepresented in services, construction, and production. The earnings and asset accumulation of the Hispanic population at large are consequently limited in comparison to that of non-Hispanic whites.

In the population at large, while 10.3% of non-Hispanic whites have household incomes below the poverty line, which for a family of four with two children was $20,444 in 2006, 24.3% of African-Americans and 20.6% of Hispanics have incomes below poverty. Poverty affects Hispanic children most seriously as

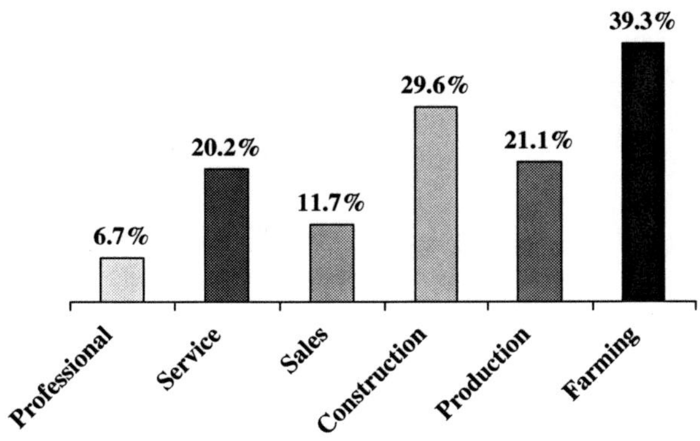

Fig. 2.10 Hispanics as a percentage of selected occupations, 2006
Source: Current Population Survey 2006.

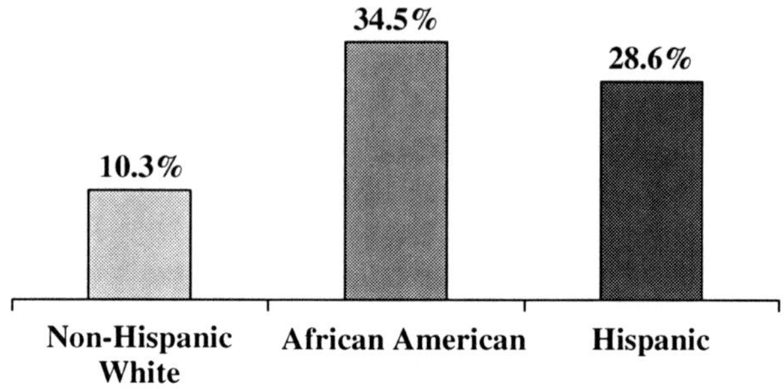

Fig. 2.11 Child poverty rate by race and Hispanic ethnicity, 2007
Source: U.S. Census Bureau (2008b).

Fig. 2.11 shows. In 2007 while 10% of non-Hispanic white children lived in families with incomes below the poverty threshold, 29% of Hispanic children lived in poverty. Low levels of human capital reduce the number of high earners among Hispanics, especially for those of Mexican origin. In 2002 while 54% of non-Hispanic white workers earned $35,000 or more, only 24% of Mexican-origin workers had incomes in this range. Approximately 35% of Cubans, Puerto Ricans, and other Hispanics had incomes this high or higher (Ramirez and de la Cruz 2003).

Low incomes translate directly into impaired asset accumulation over the life course. As we will further illustrate in Chapters 5 and 6, the situation is particularly serious for households headed by a female. Figure 2.12, which is based on a longitudinal study of individuals nearing retirement in 1992 that we will discuss further in Chapter 6, shows that while non-Hispanic white couple-headed households had over $300,000 in assets in the years just prior to retirement, Mexican-origin couple-headed households had less than $100,000 in assets. The figure clearly shows the far more serious situation for female-headed households and adds another dimension of disadvantage to that related to minority status. Figure 2.12 shows that even non-Hispanic white female-headed households had fewer assets (less than $150,000) than non-Hispanic white couple-headed household. The lack of wealth among Mexican-origin female-headed households is far more serious since they report a net worth of only $50,000. The combination of minority status and gender results in greatly exaggerated economic vulnerability. Since many children grow up

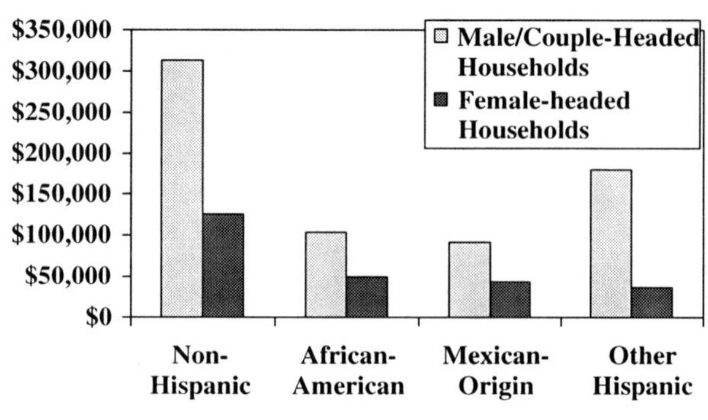

Fig. 2.12 Racial and ethnic group differences in household wealth among adults aged 51–61 years, 1992
Source: Health and Retirement Study.

in female-headed households, the low levels of income and resources contribute to the ongoing lack of educational opportunities in the Hispanic population.

These low levels of wealth among both couple-headed and female-headed households leave Hispanic families with little buffer in the event of economic crises. In the next chapter we move on to an examination of the consequences of low levels of human capital among parents for Hispanic children. As we have shown in this chapter, blocked educational opportunities translate directly into limited occupational opportunities, low wages, and the lack of work-related benefits. The result is that low-wage parents are limited in what they can do for their children and find themselves highly dependent on public programs for health care and the other services that their children need. As we will see, as important as public programs like Medicaid, cash assistance, food stamps, housing assistance, and the rest of the means-tested welfare state are, they do not fully guarantee the health and well-being of poor children.

Chapter 3
Parental Employment and Children's Security

The fact that Hispanic children are over three times more likely than non-Hispanic white children to have no health-care coverage serves as powerful testimony to the real consequences of their parent's employment vulnerability. For all groups, the lack of health insurance reduces access to care and undermines health (Children's Defense Fund 2006; Institute of Medicine 2001). The lack of health insurance, though, is only part of a package of vulnerabilities that the children of parents with low incomes and no employment benefits face. Poor and minority children are often trapped in unsafe and unhealthy neighborhoods, they suffer malnutrition in the form of diets that are high in fat, carbohydrates, and calories, and they are denied the educational opportunities that come with good schools and interaction with educationally successful peers. For children in poor neighborhoods, the streets and gang life often provide the emotional and physical security that their parents cannot provide. As we elaborate in this chapter, the long-term implications are serious for the children, their families, and for society at large.

For parents with low-paying jobs, the task of parenting can be truly challenging. As important as love and affection are in raising children, effective and successful parenting requires material resources and the ability to control the environment in which one's children grow up. Parents with steady jobs and good incomes can choose the neighborhoods in which their children live, the schools they attend, and the activities they engage in. In addition, adults with steady jobs and clear responsibilities provide important role models for their own and other children. Providing materially for one's children, represents a core adult responsibility and the inability to do so adequately adversely affects a parent's self-esteem and undermines the overall well-being of the entire family (Angel et al. 2006). The inability to provide their children adequate shelter, a good education, and recreational opportunities robs a parent of an important source of self-esteem.

A parent's employment vulnerability, then, has complex and negative emotional, behavioral, physical, and social consequences for children that have larger social implications. Inadequate health coverage, for example, undermines the health of individuals, families, and entire communities and adversely affects the productivity of the future work force (Institute of Medicine 2001, 2002, 2003a, b). The challenges faced by parents with low-wage jobs with no benefits, clearly illustrate the problems inherent in an employment-based welfare system with a publicly funded

R.J. Angel, J.L. Angel, *Hispanic Families at Risk*, DOI 10.1007/978-1-4419-0474-4_3,

social welfare safety net. As we demonstrate in this chapter, because their parents are more likely than the parents of non-Hispanic white children to have jobs that pay poorly and do not offer benefits such as health insurance, Hispanic children are particularly dependent on publicly funded programs.

Economic Vulnerability and Children's Well-Being

Even in good economic times the children of Hispanic parents are more likely than non-Hispanic children to live in subsidized housing, to receive food stamps, and to rely on Medicaid and SCHIP. In economic downturns their vulnerability increases disproportionately, as low-skilled and low-wage workers are particularly hard hit. During the first quarter of 2008, the unemployment rate for Hispanics increased to 6.5% due mainly to a slump in the construction industry, above the 4.7% rate for all non-Hispanics (Kochhar 2008). Given that the economic recession only deepened thereafter, unemployment rates will no doubt continue to increase further. The increase in unemployment is particularly serious for the foreign born, for whom the unemployment rate was 7.5% during the first quarter of 2008 as economic conditions were worsening (Kochhar 2008). Over 14% of the labor force is Hispanic and one-half of working-age Hispanics are immigrants. The rise in unemployment among Hispanics and the potential damage that a long recession could do to their already limited resource base pose serious problems for the future (Thomas et al. 2006).

Rising unemployment rates among Hispanics increase their need for publicly funded programs, such as food stamps, Medicaid, and SCHIP (Dorn et al. 2009). Unfortunately, a large fraction of children who qualify for public programs on the basis of their parents low earnings do not participate (Angel et al. 2006). Given the importance of education, good nutrition, a safe environment, and medical care to optimal development, this failure of the safety net compounds the failure of the employment-based social welfare system. In order to illustrate the unique vulnerability of Hispanic children, we review data on their family incomes, their educational experiences, their housing situations, their nutritional and income supports, their access to health care, and more. The picture we draw is one of elevated dependency on public programs as a result of their parent's low incomes and lack of access to family health insurance.

We draw upon data from various sources including a recently completed study of the lives of families in poverty and their response to welfare reform in Boston, Chicago, and San Antonio (Winston et al. 1999). We begin our examination, though, with data from the, 2007 Current Population Survey (CPS) in order to document the elevated levels of poverty among employed Hispanic and African-American families. Figure 3.1 shows the dramatic differences in poverty between minority and non-Hispanic white families in which the head of household works full time. While only 4% of non-Hispanic white working families fall below the poverty threshold, which in 2007 was $21,027 for a family of four with two children, 17% of Hispanic

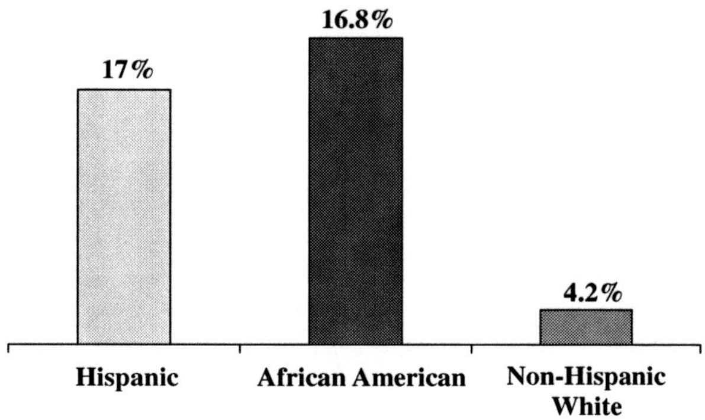

Fig. 3.1 Poverty status among American working families by race and Hispanic ethnicity, 2007
Source: Current Population Survey (2008a)

families and 16.8% of African-American families fall below the threshold. Work, and even full-time work, then is no guarantee that a minority family will not be poor.

The Earned Income Tax Credit

One of the most important income support programs for working families is the Earned Income Tax credit (EITC). This program which began during the Nixon Administration as an alternative to a negative income tax and which has been expanded several times since then provides a tax refund for poor working families (Holt 2006; National Council of La Raza 2000). In order to receive the refund, one must be a US citizen, a legal resident, or be married to a US citizen or legal resident and filing a joint tax return. Although childless couples can qualify for a small credit, the program is most generous for families with qualifying children. A family receives a tax refund based on income up to a maximum after which the refund decreases at a set rate. In 2007, the maximum refund for a family with one child was $2,853; for a family with two children the maximum refund was $4,716. The size of the refund for families with children is substantial and makes the EITC one of the nation's most important antipoverty programs. The wide support for the program results from the fact that it is based on employment and is not a direct welfare transfer.

Unfortunately, not all families with incomes low enough to qualify apply for the refund (Maag 2005). Figure 3.2 presents data from a 1999 study, one of the few available that focuses on Hispanics, comparing knowledge of and use of EITC among Hispanics with household incomes below 200% of poverty (Phillips 2001). The figure reveals rather large differences in both knowledge and use of EITC between Hispanics and non-Hispanics, as well as among Hispanics based on nativity and citizenship status. While over 75% of non-Hispanic families with incomes below 200% of poverty were aware of EITC, only 53.2% of native-born Hispanics, 29.6% of naturalized Hispanics, and 16.5% of noncitizens were aware of the program. The figure shows similar disparities in the use of the program, with Hispanics

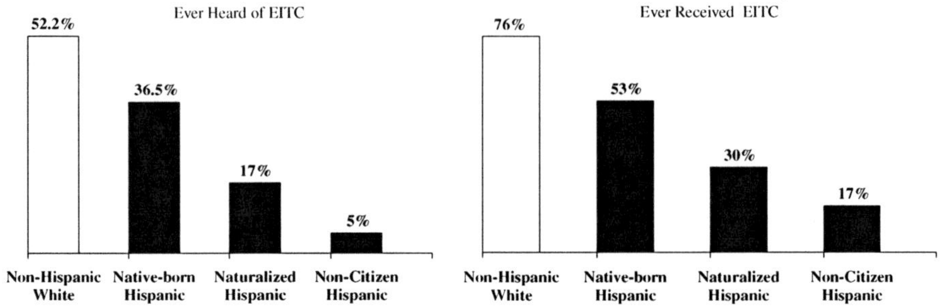

Fig. 3.2 Percentage of Hispanic families with income below 200% of poverty who ever heard of or received the earned income tax credit (EITC)
Source: 1999 National Survey of America's Families (Phillips 2001).

far less likely to actually receive EITC payments than non-Hispanic whites. The result is that although many Hispanic families are eligible for the tax credit based on their income, many fail to take advantage of the opportunity (Maag 2005; Murguía 2007). This lack of awareness has serious costs since many eligible individuals have incomes so low that they are not required to file a federal income tax form (Phillips, 2001). If they do not file and if they are not informed by some other source that they are eligible, they miss out on an important source of income.

Because of the clear importance of EITC for reducing poverty and improving the economic situations of poor families, serious outreach and information programs have been introduced since this 1999 survey was conducted. These efforts have no doubt improved participation rates among Hispanics, yet many eligible families still do not receive the tax credit. Estimates provided by the National Council of La Raza, a major advocacy organization for Hispanics, indicate that only one out of three eligible families participates (Murguía 2007). The program has other clear limitations. During times of elevated unemployment, its utility for addressing the problem of widespread poverty is reduced by the fact that it is an employment-based approach. Individuals with no earnings during the year do not qualify and must rely on other sources of income and other social programs to get by. Although the employment basis of EITC increases political support for the program, the fact that many eligible families and unemployed heads of household do not participate further illustrates the inherent weakness of an employment-based welfare state for minority Americans.

Public Assistance Programs

As a result of low incomes, a large number of Hispanic households, and especially those with young children, must rely on public assistance. As we have seen earlier, the Mexican-origin population not only makes up the majority of the Hispanic population but also is economically worse off than other Hispanic subgroups. In

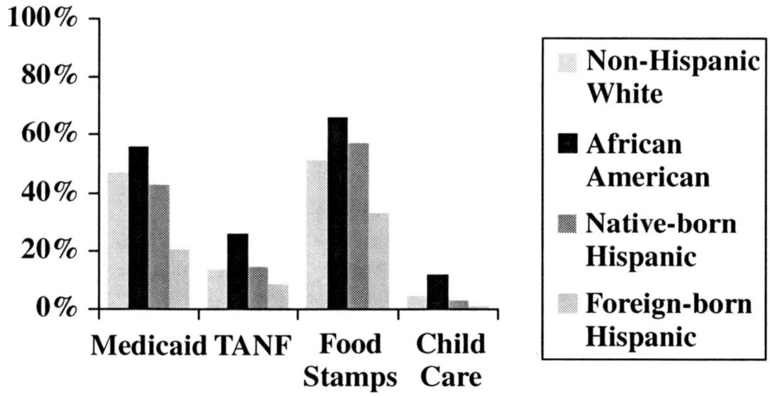

Fig. 3.3 Program participation by families with children under 5 years and household incomes less than half of the poverty threshold
Source: Current Population Survey (2004, 2006). Percentages are weighted.

order to examine patterns of public program use by Mexican-origin families, we employ a combined sample of the March *Current Population Survey*, also known as the Annual Demographic Survey, for 2004 and 2006. This combined sample provides a large-enough sample of Mexican-origin families for a detailed analysis of their use of various programs. A detailed explanation of the pooling of these multiple Annual Demographic Surveys is provided in Angel et al. (2009). Figure 3.3 provides detailed information on group differences in participation in several major public social welfare programs by different levels of the ratio of household income to poverty for non-Hispanic whites, African-Americans, and Mexican-origin families by nativity. We restrict the figure to families with at least one child less than 5 years of age. Although we have computed the same information for families in which the youngest child is older, the patterns are similar and we only discuss them briefly.

Figure 3.3 highlights several important patterns for Hispanic households with infants. At the lowest level of household income, households with incomes less than half of the poverty rate, or an income of $9,903 or lower for a family of four with two children in 2005, a substantial fraction of families of all sorts do not use Medicaid. This is a rather striking finding since at that level of poverty a family with a child under 5 years clearly qualifies. The figure also shows that only 20.4% of foreign-born Mexican-origin families use Medicaid. The combination of extreme poverty and the failure to use Medicaid has serious negative implications for the long-term health and productivity of these children.

The figure shows that African-American families are the most frequent users of all of the services listed; native-born Mexican-origin families use these services at high rates, but at rates far lower than African-Americans. For all services, and especially child care and Supplemental Security Income (SSI), foreign-born Mexican-origin families are the least likely to participate. The figure also shows that as household income goes up, program use by all groups drops and that Mexican-origin families are less likely than African-American families to use services. Again, foreign-born Mexican-origin families are the least likely to benefit from these services. Clearly, publicly funded and means-tested programs do not address the full range of needs of poor Mexican-origin families. Perhaps what is most striking is that even among poor non-Hispanic families who clearly qualify, many do not participate in the major social support programs for the poor.

Although we do not present the figures, patterns of use of these services are lower among families with children older than 5 years than among families with infants, largely because as children get older the income eligibility rules tighten. Nonetheless, even though they are lower overall, group differences in social service use by families with older children are similar to those for families with younger children. Foreign-born Mexican-origin families are the least likely to participate, even at extremely low levels of household income. Multivariate analyses that we do not present here show that differences in poverty, family size, education, marital status, age, and maternal health largely account for the difference in social service use between native-born Mexican-origin households and non-Hispanic white households. Even when we take these factors into account, though, the difference between foreign-born Mexican-origin families and non-Hispanic white families in the use of these means-tested public programs remains large and significant.

Health Insurance: Medicaid and SCHIP

Among the most important social welfare programs in any nation are those that provide health care to children. Medicaid and the State Children's Health Insurance Program (SCHIP) provide health-care coverage to poor children and children in families with incomes a good bit above the poverty threshold. As of the writing of this chapter, President Obama had just signed legislation that President Bush had twice vetoed to extend coverage under SCHIP to allow states to cover a larger number of children in families that earn too much to qualify for Medicaid. President Bush agreed with those fiscal and social conservatives who worry that overly generous public health insurance programs will undermine our employment-based system and serve as a backdoor to universal and mandatory public health insurance. Some explanation of Medicaid and SCHIP is necessary to understanding the importance of these programs for Hispanic children.

Medicaid was introduced in 1965 to provide health-care coverage to low-income parents, children, seniors, and people with disabilities (Eldridge 2007). The program is jointly funded by the federal and state governments under general guidelines that give states discretion in determining eligibility criteria and the services covered. Eligible individuals include those with low incomes and few assets who are young, very old and infirm, pregnant, disabled, or blind. Income and asset tests differ by state and the group covered. To qualify, one must also be a U.S. citizen or lawfully admitted immigrant. Although most enrollees in Medicaid are children in poor families, the majority of the funds spent are for the care of older individuals in nursing homes and the disabled (Tritz 2005).

Because of the fact that Medicaid does not cover all children in families with limited incomes, the SCHIP was introduced as part of the Balanced Budget Act of 1997. Like regular Medicaid, this is a joint federal/state program that allows states to cover children in families that do not qualify for regular Medicaid because their income is above the eligibility level. SCHIP provides block grants for states to offer coverage to children either by extending their regular Medicaid programs to children who do not qualify for regular Medicaid, or by creating a new program not directly tied to regular Medicaid, or by developing some sort of combined program. States retain considerable discretion in the structure of their Medicaid programs (Smith and Rousseau 2005). Every state now has an approved SCHIP program and the initiative has been a clear success in extending coverage to more families (Center for Children and Families 2007). The program had broad initial support and retains it today, largely because it is paid for by a "sin tax" on tobacco products.

Between 1998 and 2007, Congress authorized $40 billion to support the program. When SCHIP was signed into law, there were an estimated 11.5 million uninsured children in the United States (Centers for Medicare and Medicaid Services 1999). Of those, 4.2 million were eligible for coverage under Medicaid and approximately 2.4 million more became eligible for SCHIP (Eisert and Gabow 2002). Since 1997, the number of uninsured low-income children in the United States has decreased by one-third. Today the program covers more than 7 million individuals including low-income pregnant women and parents (Congressional Budget Office 2007; Schwarz et al. 2007). However, the number of uninsured children continues to rise, largely because many children still do not meet income eligibility criteria (Schwarz et al. 2007). Hopefully the expansion that President Obama has signed into law will allow SCHIP to cover even more children.

Despite the program's success, new strategies are required in order to more effectively reach the two-thirds of children who currently qualify for SCHIP or Medicaid coverage and yet are not enrolled (Broaddus and Ku 2000). Outreach is particularly important in reaching Hispanic children, again especially those in Mexican-origin families. An examination of the use of the role of Medicaid and SCHIP in providing health care to individuals in families facing serious economic hardship makes it clear that these programs form the basis of whatever health-care security poor families have (National Council of La Raza 2008).

Private Employment-Based Health Coverage

Because of the high cost of providing health insurance plans to their employees, many employers are shifting a larger fraction of the cost onto employees, with the result that a larger number of workers find coverage too expensive (Agency for Healthcare Research and Quality 2005; Long and Shen 2004). As a result, the proportion of Americans covered by private plans has been decreasing (U.S. Census

Bureau 2005). A summary of recent trends in sources of health-care coverage compiled by *Child Trends* illustrates this shift in coverage for children in the United States. Between 2000 and 2003, the percentage of all children under 18 years with private health insurance coverage decreased from 71 to 66%. At the same time, the percentage of children enrolled in Medicaid increased from 20 to 26% (Child Trends Data Bank 2003). Unfortunately, as the number of children in families with no private health insurance increases, a large fraction of children who qualify for public coverage because their family's income is low are not participating in Medicaid or SCHIP (Dubay et al. 2002; Guyer 2000; Perry et al. 2000).

Part of the increase in the number of the uninsured can be attributed to the fact that a growing fraction of workers are employed in jobs that do not offer health-care coverage (Long and Shen 2004; Shen and Zuckerman 2003). In recent years the proportion of workers employed in services has increased at the same time that employment in manufacturing has decreased. In addition, a growing fraction of workers are working part time or for small firms that do not have the employee base to negotiate favorable group health plans (Long and Shen 2004). Although these changes affect all groups and are increasing the employment and social benefit in security of a large faction of Americans, they affect Hispanics disproportionately. Low levels of education and few job skills represent serious health-care coverage vulnerabilities. One particularly vulnerable group that many would exclude from the receipt of social services altogether is noncitizens and their children (Chollet 1994).

One serious consequence of the lack of insurance that was revealed in a study we conducted among poor families in Boston, Chicago, and San Antonio was that many poor families accumulate massive medical debt that they can never realistically pay off and that becomes a serious economic burden that makes it almost impossible to save (Angel et al. 2006). Another consequence of the lack of a group-sponsored family plan was that in many families very ill parents spent much effort to obtain Medicaid for their children while simply giving up on finding the medical care they needed for themselves, and in other cases some children in the family, usually the younger ones, were covered by Medicaid while their older siblings had no coverage (Angel and Lein 2006).

Table 3.1 presents detailed information on the sources of health-care coverage for children and adolescents under 18 years in non-Hispanic white, African-American, and Hispanic families. In order to illustrate the serious disadvantage among Mexican-origin Hispanics, we present the data separately for three Hispanic subgroups. The table shows that Hispanic children are less likely than non-Hispanic white children to have private health-care coverage, a category that consists overwhelmingly of employment-based coverage. What stands out starkly is the very low coverage among Mexican-origin children and adolescents; fewer than 40% have private coverage. Very few children are covered by the military. In the absence of private coverage, the fallback is Medicaid and indeed the table reveals higher rates of Medicaid use by Hispanics and African-Americans than by non-Hispanic whites. Medicaid, though, does not make up for the lack of private coverage. The last row shows very high proportions of children with no coverage at all. Even among non-Hispanic whites over 7% of parents report that their children have no coverage

Table 3.1 Health-care coverage from major sources for non-Hispanic whites African-Americans and three Hispanic groups by age for children 0–17 years (unweighted *N*s in parentheses), 2006

Type of coverage	Non-Hispanic white	African-American	Mexican origin	Cuban-American	Puerto Rican
Private (%)	78.2	48.4	38.7	60.0	46.2
Medicare (%)	0.4	1.5	0.7	1.4	0.7
Medicaid (%)	17.8	44.1	40.6	25.4	46.7
Champ (%)	3.2	2.9	1.4	0	4.2
None (%)	7.2	13.1	23.6	18.2	10.3
Total (*N*)	(78,657)	(14,049)	16,590	590	2,505

Source: Current Population Survery (2004, 2006)

at all. The situation is clearly most serious among those of Mexican origin, though, over 23% of whom have no coverage. The situation is particularly serious in Texas in which 35% of the population is of Mexican origin.

As in many of the other areas we have discussed, immigrants are at particularly high risk of lacking health-care coverage, (Angel and Angel 2007). Researchers have found that immigration status has a profound effect on Medicaid participation. In one study researchers found that 5% of Mexican immigrant workers in industries that do not rely heavily on Mexican immigrants are covered by Medicaid and other public insurance (Wallace 2007). These same researchers report that over two-thirds of Mexican immigrants are employed in types of jobs that are heavily reliant on Mexican immigrants but offer no medical coverage.

The picture that emerges then is one of a serious lack of health-care coverage among Mexican-origin children and especially among immigrant families. The unique vulnerability of this population has been frequently documented and many have asked why it occurs. There appears to be no clear answer and many factors contribute to the problem. Language and administrative barriers clearly contribute. The Three-City Study clearly documented the complexity of the application process for public coverage and the difficulty parents often have in understanding the requirements. Official policy is clearly one potential cause of differential coverage rates. Although Medicaid operates under general federal guidelines and are required to offer a minimal package of services to needy infants and children, states retain a great deal of discretion in terms of application procedures, income requirements, and benefit amounts.

One of the major reasons for the large number of uninsured children in the United States is that many children in poor families are not enrolled (Selden et al. 1998). Differences in state eligibility criteria, as well as local administration of the program, are of major importance in determining who enrolls (Angel et al. 2006). The study of poor families in Boston, Chicago, and San Antonio that we mentioned above provides some useful insights into the role of state policies on the extent of health-care coverage among poor children. Boston, Chicago, and San Antonio have very diverse populations, but they are also located in states with very different welfare policies (Winston et al. 1999). Texas has traditionally provided very little more than what is required under federal law, Massachusetts has provided a generous package of services, and Illinois has been somewhere between the two in terms of generosity.

In addition to other information, the study determined the extent and sources of health-care coverage among poor families and Table 3.2 provides very revealing information concerning state differences in Medicaid coverage of children in families with low incomes. The table shows the proportion of children who participate in Medicaid for different levels of the ratio of family income to poverty. The first row, shows that in Boston and Chicago, 82% of children in families with incomes below 100% of poverty are covered by Medicaid. In Texas, though, only 64% of children in families with incomes below 100% of poverty are enrolled in Medicaid. Much lower rates of participation in Texas could reflect the fact that many Mexican-origin families do not participate even though they qualify. To some extent, though, they reflect state differences in administration, funding, and outreach. State differences in eligibility become even more salient as one moves up in income. The last row of Table 3.2 shows that among families with incomes just below 200% of the poverty threshold, while 64% of children are covered by Medicaid in Boston, only 5% are covered in Texas. Illinois is intermediate, clearly revealing the importance of state differences in Medicaid policy as well as in population composition.

Table 3.2 Children covered by Medicaid

Family income relative to federal poverty (%)	All three cities (%)	Boston (%)	Chicago (%)	San Antonio (%)	March 2000 CPS (%)
<100	77	82	82	64	60
100–124	58	86	59	30	42
125–149	53	63	61	35	33
150–199	34	64	35	5	23

In order to determine whether population composition is primarily responsible for these state differences, we performed a multivariate analysis to control for population composition. Hispanics in San Antonio are primarily of Mexican origin, so one might ask if the lower rates of coverage in Texas reflect the fact that the state's poor population is disproportionately of Mexican origin. In each Three-City Study household, extensive information was collected on one randomly selected "focal" child. The analysis we performed, but do not present here because of their complexity, examined the probability that the focal child would have any insurance and whether he or she was covered by Medicaid. The results were rather dramatic and reveal that even when other factors are controlled, Mexican-origin children are only 29% as likely to be covered by any form of health insurance and 43% as likely to be covered by Medicaid as non-Mexican Hispanics.

The analyses revealed other interesting associations that reflect national and state policy related to health-care coverage. Although mother's citizenship status did not predict the probability of a child having health insurance of some sort, the children of mothers who were US citizens were only 59% as likely as those whose mothers are not citizens to receive Medicaid. This may reflect the fact that immigrants are more dependent on public health coverage than native-born families. On the other hand, the child's own citizenship status greatly influenced the probability that he or she would be covered by some form of health insurance. Children born in the United States were far more likely to have health insurance, including Medicaid, than noncitizen children. Most public programs base eligibility on US citizenship, so this finding is to be expected (Zambrana and Logie 2000). The multivariate analyses also revealed that children in San Antonio were less than half as likely as children in Boston to be covered by any form of health insurance and only 60% as likely to be covered by Medicaid.

The Future of Our Nation

Children are our future and the fact that in the future a large fraction of the population will be minority means that we will be living in a very different country, as will the nations of Europe. By 2042 minority Americans will make up the majority of the population (U.S. Census Bureau 2008a). As we have noted, that increase will have particular implications for the labor force in the not so distant future. The labor force of the twenty-first century will be largely Hispanic and their level of productivity will determine the material quality of life for everyone. As we note, in 1945 there were 50 workers supporting each retired person (Social Security Administration 2004a). Today that number has shrunk to three and in the future it will drop even lower (Social Security Administration 2004b), meaning that nearly half of those contributing to Social Security, national defense, education, infrastructure, and the rest of what makes up civilization will be Hispanic. Given their high rates of immigration and the demographic inertia inherent in a youthful population with high fertility rates, a large fraction of that group will be of Mexican origin.

The major recession that began in 2008 and that brought serious economic hardship to all nations of the world resulted in major deficits and the need to curtail government spending. At a time when the need for universal health coverage in the United States had been accepted by almost all parties, the economic crises raises new questions as to how to pay for it. As the baby-boom generation begins to reach 65 years in 2011, the fiscal burden caused by massive deficit spending and growing Social Security and Medicare expenditures will require significant budgetary constraints. This fact will inevitably result in a contentious debate concerning the sources of savings. Given the relative political weakness of minority groups who have few connections to the worlds of economic or political power, the competition for resources may result in major harm to the most vulnerable. Given the fact that the economy will be heavily dependent on Hispanic workers, it is imperative that the educational levels of this population, and especially their mastery of mathematics and science, be greatly and rapidly enhanced. In addition, in order for the labor force of the future to be as productive as will be necessary, the health of its members must be excellent. Cuts in educational programs and health-care programs for poor minority children are seriously self-destructive for the United States as a whole. As Marta Tienda puts it, "Realizing the demographic dividend afforded by the infusion of young Hispanics into an aging white society requires lowering poverty rates, closing achievement gaps, and raising college enrollment and graduation rates" (Tienda 2007; p. 32).

In this chapter we have documented the serious vulnerability of children in Hispanic households and identified specific characteristics that increase that vulnerability. Today, a huge fraction of Hispanic as well as African-American children are growing up in poverty and have inferior educational opportunities and less than optimal health care (Reimers 2006). If children are our future, that future does not seem bright. We mentioned some of the major safety net programs and showed how state policies related to Medicaid can affect the well-being of children. These programs are vital to the health and well-being of minority children, but they are insufficient. Expanding them will be very difficult in the period of serious fiscal constraint that we have entered and that may well be permanent. The result is that we may not be able to count on economic growth to finance the health, educational, and family support programs that are necessary for our collective economic survival. In such an environment, political discourse and actions will have to deal with very difficult issues of redistribution and the ways in which the aggregate pie is distributed.

Chapter 4
Employment and Benefits for Working-Age Hispanic Males

In the last chapter we showed that children's economic, social, and health-care vulnerabilities result directly from their parent's lack of an adequate income and job benefits, including access to employment-based group health plans. In the next two chapters we will look closely at the occupational situations of those parents as well as of childless Hispanic males and females. In this chapter we examine the issue of access to work-related benefits among Hispanic males, with a special focus on Mexican-origin males. As we have shown in previous chapters, the Mexican-origin population is not only the largest segment of the Hispanic population but also the most disadvantaged in terms of employment benefits. Even among those who are employed full-time full-year, Mexican-origin workers earn less than non-Hispanic whites and have low rates of retirement and health-care coverage. In order to identify the sources of these disadvantages we examine the types of jobs in which Mexican-origin men are employed.

The US labor force is highly stratified and the best jobs, including professional and managerial positions, are disproportionately held by non-Hispanic white males (Bean and Bell-Rose 1999; Borjas 1990; Borjas and Katz 2007; Kochhar 2005; Tienda and Mitchell 2006b; Toussaint-Comeau 2004). Hispanics, along with African-Americans, are confined to lower paying, less-prestigious occupations (Bean and Bell-Rose 1999). As we will show, they are concentrated in specific occupational sectors including agriculture, construction, and services in which salaries are low and benefits rare (Angel et al. 2009). This concentration in low-benefit sectors may represent a major reason for the income and benefit disadvantage that we document, and in this chapter we explore this possibility. If such sectoral ghettoization is a major reason for low rates of coverage among Mexican-origin male workers, we would expect to find that within sectors, rates of coverage for African-American and non-Hispanic white male workers are similar to those for Mexican-origin workers. If rates of coverage are lower for Mexican-origin workers than for African-American or non-Hispanic workers even within sectors or more refined occupational categories, then factors unique to Mexican origin must be involved.

In Chapter 2 we reviewed the theory of segmented assimilation, which refers to a process by which certain immigrant families move into the middle class within one or two generations, while others remain trapped in lower classes even after several generations. Available data suggest that this difference is influenced by an

R.J. Angel, J.L. Angel, *Hispanic Families at Risk*, DOI 10.1007/978-1-4419-0474-4_4,

immigrant's initial human capital endowment, specifically his or her English language proficiency and education. Occupational differences between immigrants and non-Hispanic whites and native-born Hispanics decrease over time for those who are more fluent in English and have higher levels of education (Bean and Tienda 1990; Kochhar 2005; Stolzenberg 1990; Toussaint-Comeau 2004). Unfortunately, because they have very little education and are often only marginally fluent in English, Mexican-origin immigrants face particularly serious challenges to economic mobility (Tienda and Mitchell 2006a). Individual characteristics, then, probably interact with occupational structure in complex ways to affect the long-term mobility chances of Mexican-origin men. Whatever the mechanisms that give rise to the vulnerability of this population, though, it is indisputable that a large fraction of Mexican-origin families remain in the lower classes even after generations in the United States.

Many studies find that employment in low-wage sectors of the economy in which benefits are not offered is one of the most important reasons for the difference in benefit coverage between Hispanics and the general population (Schur and Feldman 2000). But other occupational factors are important as well. One critically important characteristic of the firms in which Hispanics tend to be employed relates to their size (Schur and Feldman 2000). Small firms are less likely than larger firms to offer retirement coverage or group health plans simply because they are less able to afford them. Later we provide evidence that within occupational categories Mexican-origin male workers are more likely than non-Hispanic workers to be employed in small firms. Such firms are more vulnerable than larger firms to economic downturns and employment in small firms may be associated not only with a lack of benefits but also with greater employment insecurity and more frequent layoffs.

It is possible, of course, that low rates of participation in company-sponsored retirement and group health plans by Mexican-origin and other Hispanic workers are the worker's choice. When such plans are voluntary some employees choose not to participate, especially when they are young. Even among workers with above-average incomes, a significant percentage do not have health insurance (Fronstin 2005b; Huynh et al. 2006). In the United States, participation in retirement and health plans, other than Social Security and Medicare, is not mandatory and although many employers automatically enroll new employees in such plans, many do not. When such plans are offered on a voluntary basis, the employee has the option of participating or not and some choose not to.

Employment Characteristics

Hispanic males, including those of Mexican origin, are by and large employed (Bureau of Labor Statistics 2008). Yet since the economic crisis began in 2008 their employment situation has deteriorated along with that of the rest of the labor force. In January 2008 before the recession decimated the economy, the unemployment rate for Hispanic males 20 years and older was 6.2%. By January 2009 it had climbed to 11% (Bureau of Labor Statistics 2009a). Given the continuing deterioration of the global economy, the unemployment rate among Hispanics is bound to increase. Yet as high as current official unemployment rates are for all groups, they probably seriously underestimate the actual fraction of the population that is unemployed, especially for minority groups. Official unemployment estimates are based on the government's definition of the labor force. In order to be classified as unemployed, one must be counted as a member of the labor force.

The labor force consists of individuals who are currently employed and those who are unemployed but who have looked for work at some time during the 4 weeks preceding the survey in which information on employment is collected (Bureau of Labor Statistics 2001). This definition excludes individuals who have not looked for work during the preceding 4 weeks and those who have given up on the possibility of finding a job. After months of fruitless job hunting some individuals simply give up. The number of discouraged workers increases in economic downturns when jobs become scarce. Estimates by the Department of Labor indicate the number of discouraged workers increased between 2008, when the recession began, and 2009 (Bureau of Labor Statistics 2009b). When examining labor force statistics it is important to keep the discouraged worker phenomenon in mind, especially when dealing with groups that are highly vulnerable to long-term unemployment. As in other parts of the world, when formal employment is not available individuals enter the informal economy and earn money as they can. It is impossible to know the extent to which that might be occurring in the United States today.

Official employment and unemployment statistics mask another important phenomenon that undermines the economic security of Hispanics and other minority Americans. Many individuals who need full-time employment can only find part-time work, or their employers have cut their hours because of slow demand (Stoddard 2008). In addition, many jobs are seasonal and others, including many in construction in which Hispanics are concentrated, are by definition temporary and when a worker is not working he earns nothing (Lazo 2008). Middle-class workers with a salary can count on a steady and predictable income; low-wage workers who work on an hourly basis cannot. Their income fluctuates with the amount of work that is available. In economic downturns many employers have no choice but to reduce hours, even when they do not let someone go completely.

Whatever the real employment rate is, though, for all racial and cultural groups the norm is for men to work. A male's worth as a person is determined by his ability to fulfill his responsibilities toward his family and children. Most men, therefore, do what they can to generate whatever income they are able to. Clearly, some resort to illegal activities because of either character flaws or desperation, but the vast majority attempt to find and keep legitimate employment. Unfortunately, even when they do find work, Hispanic males do not earn the same as non-Hispanic white or African-American males. Figure 4.1 shows that among full-time workers the average weekly wage is $879 for non-Hispanic white males and $683 for African-American males, but only $595 for Hispanic males. This serious salary deficit no doubt reflects the limited educational backgrounds of Hispanic men that we documented earlier, but it also reflects other factors that we investigate below.

Figure 4.1 Hispanic male workers earn less per week than non-Hispanic whites and blacks (in dollars), 2007
Source: Bureau of Labor Statistics (2008).

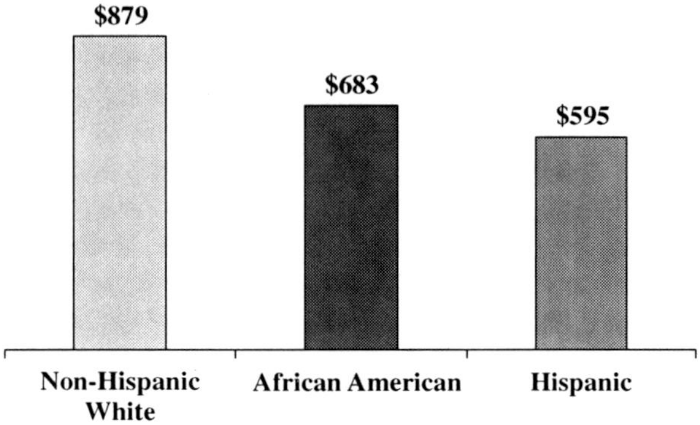

Figure 4.2 Occupational distribution of male workforce of Hispanics and non-Hispanic whites, 2007
Source: Bureau of Labor Statistics (2008).

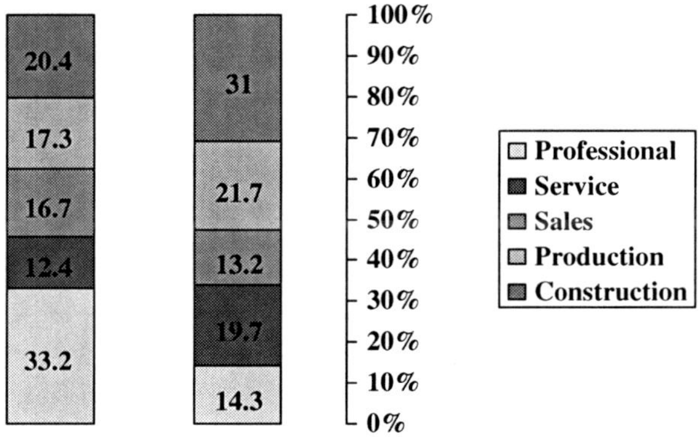

Figure 4.2 presents the occupational distribution of Hispanic and non-Hispanic white male workers among five occupational categories. These stack graphs show that Hispanic males are far less likely than non-Hispanic males to be employed in professional occupations. While 33.2% of employed non-Hispanic white men are professionals, only 14.3% of employed Hispanic men are professionals. One the other hand, far higher percentages of Hispanic than non-Hispanic white males are employed in production, construction, and services. Again, this distribution reflects at least in part the lower educational levels among Hispanics, but it clearly means that the population as a whole does not share the earnings potential of non-Hispanic whites. We suspect that even within the category of professional, Hispanic males do not occupy the highest positions with the most economic and political power. Few reach the highest offices in public life. At the time we were writing this book Mel Martinez of Florida was planning on retiring from the US Senate in 2010 and Ken Salazar of Colorado resigned to accept the position of Interior Secretary, leaving Robert Menendez of New Jersey as the only Hispanic member of the US Senate (Navarrette 2009).

Retirement Coverage

With an examination of aspects of employment and income as introduction, we now move on to an examination of retirement and health insurance coverage among Hispanic males. We then return to a closer examination of the employment situation of Mexican-origin males to complete our analysis. As we have suggested, employment in the sectors in which Hispanics are concentrated and especially when they are employed in small firms and in lower paid positions are probably major reasons for low rates of retirement and health-care coverage. Let us examine this possibility further. In Fig. 4.3, we present data from the 2006 Current Population Survey (CPS) to document the low retirement plan participation rates among men 25–64 years old by race and Mexican origin. Here retirement plans include private pensions and annuities, government employment pensions, Railroad Retirement, and individual Keogh and 401(k) plans. As the figure reveals, Mexican-origin workers are half as likely as non-Hispanic whites and African-Americans to have any private retirement plan.

Figure 4.3 Any pension coverage for men aged 25–64 years, 2006
Source: Current Population Survey (2004, 2006).

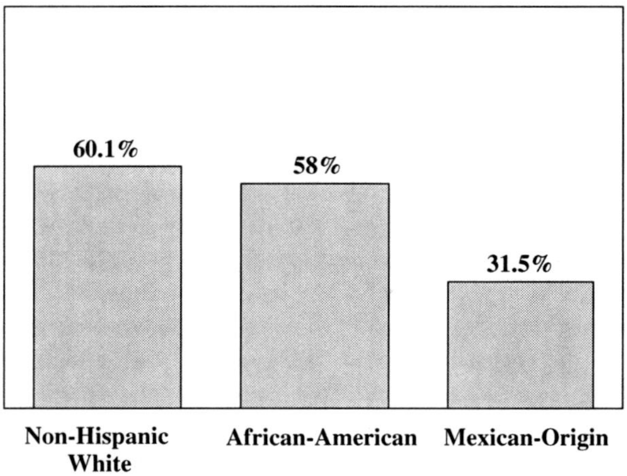

The fact that Mexican-origin men have such low rates of retirement coverage represents a serious problem for the economic security of the group as a whole. Older individuals who are unable to work and who have inadequate incomes either do without the health care and basic necessities they need or they become a drain on their families. Yet this low level of formal retirement coverage masks another problem that accompanies the general shift from defined-benefit to defined-contribution plans. Defined-benefit plans guarantee a worker a set income for life based on some formula related to the length of his or her employment and highest wage (Munnell and Sundén 2004). These plans also include an incentive for early retirement since even with a lower prorated payment, the lifetime payout is higher than it would be if a worker continued on until 65 years. In short, there is little reason to continue working past 62 when currently most men retire. Defined-contribution plans do not guarantee a set income and one's retirement security depends on what one saves during one's working years. The incentive for early retirement is also lower since the longer one works, the more one saves. Most workers, unfortunately, do not save enough even with an employer contribution to assure a secure income for several years (Munnell and Sundén 2004).

The economic downturn of 2008 underscores the real danger that the investments on which 401(k) plans are based can lose real value. Most workers have seen the value of their 401(k) plans drop by huge amounts, which seriously compounds the problem that so many were underfunded to begin with (Laise 2009). Again the situation is particularly serious for Hispanics among whom participation in employer-based 401(k) plans is half that of the general population. The average balance in those accounts is less than one-fifth that of the overall workforce, \$10,480 for Hispanics compared to \$53,670 for the population at large (Orszag and Rodriguez 2005). The economic downturn has greatly eroded the value of 401(k) plans generally leaving even Hispanic workers who are lucky enough to have a retirement plan with even less to live on in retirement.

Health Insurance

The data, then, clearly reveal a serious deficiency among Hispanics in retirement income security. Jobs that do not provide retirement benefits are unlikely to pay well enough to allow a worker to save and invest for retirement. The higher fertility and larger families typical of Hispanics mean that their limited earnings must be used for daily consumption, which leaves little left to save. When asked if they feel that they are saving enough for retirement, nearly half of working Hispanics report that they are not (Holley 2006). Low levels of savings and wealth mean that the medical expenses that accompany aging present a serious financial risk. In one study, one of every seven older respondents reported that paying medical bills was either very difficult or that it had used up all their savings (Schoen et al. 1998). Medical debt is one of the leading causes of bankruptcy for both younger and older adults (Gurewich et al. 2004; Himmelstein et al. 2005; Jacoby et al. 2001). Even with Medicare, medical expenses can represent a serious drain on a retired household's income and assets (Daschle et al. 2008). The expenses that Medicare does not pay, such as those for some medical appliances, in addition to the premium for Part B, co-payments, and cost sharing for hospitalizations, can result in significant debt (Gurewich et al. 2004).

Health-care expenses, then, are clearly a potential major source of debt among retirees, but health care is something one needs throughout life and group health insurance represents a major work-related benefit. We again turn to the CPS to obtain a large-enough sample of Mexican-origin men to examine group differences in health insurance coverage. In order to obtain this large sample, we employ the combined 2004 and 2006 March CPS, also known as the Annual Social and Economic Supplement (ASEC) (Angel et al. 2009). The ASEC is particularly useful for our purposes because it includes a large oversample of Mexican-origin workers.

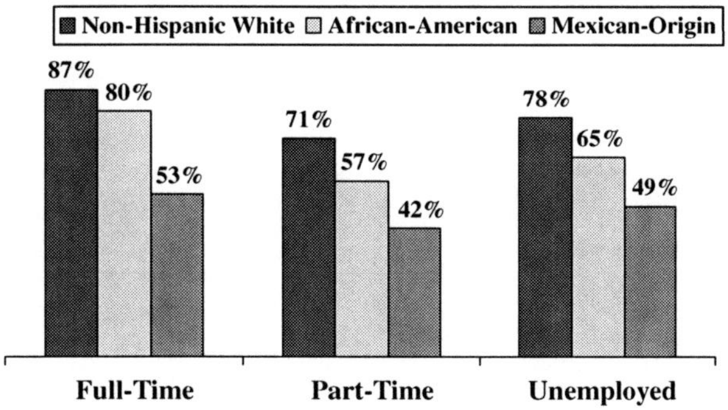

Figure 4.4 Percentage of males aged 18–64 years with insurance by employment status, 2006
Source: Current Population Survey (2004, 2006).

Figure 4.4 presents the percentage of non-Hispanic, Mexican-origin, and African-American men, 18–64 years old, with health insurance coverage by their employment status. The figure excludes full-time students and members of the armed forces. It reveals that Mexican-origin men are far less likely than either non-Hispanic white or African-American men to have health insurance regardless of their employment status. Non-Hispanic white males who are employed full time have the highest rates of coverage, and although full-time employed African-American men have lower rates than non-Hispanic white men they are far more likely to have coverage than full-time employed Mexican-origin males, nearly half of whom are not covered. Even among the unemployed, coverage is much higher for non-Hispanic white and African-American men than for Mexican-origin men. These relatively high rates of coverage among the currently unemployed to a large extent reflect coverage from a previous employer. Among those men who reported that they were currently unemployed in this sample, 52% of non-Hispanic whites, 31% of African-Americans, but only 27% of Mexican-origin respondents reported that they had employer-provided health insurance coverage at some point during the past year. A smaller fraction had coverage through a spouse, 18.4% of non-Hispanic white men, 15.7% of African-American men, and 9.1% of Mexican-origin men. This table, therefore, makes it clear that the overall lower rates of coverage among Mexican-origin men do not result from a greater likelihood of unemployment. Their rate of coverage is far lower than that of non-Hispanics even among those employed full time.

In Table 4.1 we restrict the analysis to employed men and examine their employment characteristics in greater detail in order to get some idea of the sorts of jobs Mexican-origin men hold compared with non-Hispanic white or African-American men. In this and the following tables we focus on health coverage from employment or a union. Table 4.1 again shows high rates of employment for all groups. To begin to compare the employment experiences of these three groups of men and relate those to their access to benefits, we begin by examining where they are employed in terms of large occupational sectors or categories, as well as their union membership. We begin by distinguishing between those employed in the public and private sectors, as well as the self-employed. The public sector includes jobs in local, state,

Table 4.1 Employment Sector Characteristics of Employed Men by Race and Mexican Origin

Characteristic	Non-Hispanic White	Mexican-Origin	African American
Employment Hours (%)			
Fulltime[b]	93.3	93.9	91.1
Employment Sector (%)			
Private	72.7	87.2	76.9
Public	12.4	6.1	17.0
Self-employed	14.9	6.8	6.1
Union Membership (%)	15.6	10.1	19.6
Occupation (%)			
Management	15.2	4.5	6.3
Business and financial operations	4.1	1.1	2.8
Computer and mathematical sciences	3.3	0.8	2.4
Architecture and engineering	3.7	0.7	1.9
Life, physical, and social sciences	1.2	0.2	0.7
Community and social service	1.1	0.5	2.1
Legal	1.3	0.2	0.5
Education, training and library	3.3	1.1	2.5
Arts, design, entertainment, sports, media	2.0	1.0	1.7
Healthcare practitioner and technical	2.6	0.7	2.0
Healthcare support	0.3	0.3	1.1
Public safety, protective service	3.0	1.8	5.6
Food preparation and serving	2.4	8.6	4.8
Building and grounds cleaning, maintenance	2.7	9.0	6.1
Personal care and service	0.9	0.8	2.3
Sales	11.9	6.5	6.9
Office and administrative support	5.6	5.5	9.6
Farming, fishing and forestry	0.7	3.7	0.6
Construction and extraction	10.7	23.1	7.7
Installation, maintenance and repair	7.3	6.0	5.2
Production	8.5	13.1	10.9
Transportation and material moving	8.5	11.2	16.5
Firm Size (%)			
Less than 10 employees	23.1	24.6	13.8
10–24	9.4	15.7	7.4
25–99	13.2	17.5	12.8
100 or more	54.3	42.3	66.0
Firm Size Excluding Self-Employed (%)			
Less than 10 employees	12.1	19.9	8.9
10–24	9.7	16.5	7.5
25–99	14.8	18.5	13.5
100 or more	63.4	45.1	70.1
N	63,834	9,729	7,264

Source: Current Population Survey, 2004, 2006

and federal governments, most of which offer benefits. State and local government workers are highly concentrated in the education sector and include teachers and university professors (Employee Benefit Research Institute 2005). The public sector also has a relatively high unionization rate. The private sector category includes all small and large private firms; the self-employed category includes self-employed service sector workers such as doctors and lawyers in private practice, independent contractors, and individuals who mow lawns or perform small-scale domestic services. These broad categories, then, include very different jobs, but they serve to begin our examination of the occupational distribution of the Mexican-origin population.

Table 4.1 reveals large differences among the three groups of men in terms of these broad employment sectors. Compared with non-Hispanic white and African-American males, Mexican-origin males are less likely to be employed in the public sector, in which African-Americans have the highest representation. Mexican-origin males, like African-American males, are also less likely than non-Hispanic males to be self-employed and as we will see within the self-employed category they hold low-paying and low-prestige positions. Relatively few are doctors, lawyers, or advanced degree independent contractors with high incomes. Table 4.1 also shows that Mexican-origin males are less likely than the other two groups to belong to a union, a characteristic that again reduces their access to health insurance and retirement plans. Historically, union membership has been a major source of coverage for American workers (Hirsch et al. 1997).

Table 4.1 provides yet more insight into the source of benefit vulnerability among Mexican-origin workers. Only 4.5% of the Mexican-origin sample holds management positions, a rate below that of either non-Hispanic whites or African-Americans. On the other hand, 23.1% of the Mexican-origin sample is employed in construction and 9% is employed in building and grounds care. The data, then, begin to present an occupational profile for Mexican-origin males that includes jobs in sectors of the economy with low rates of health insurance as well as retirement coverage.

It begins to appear then the low rates of benefit coverage among Mexican-origin males may result from their unfavorable occupational distribution or other characteristics of the jobs they hold. One possibility is that they are employed in small firms which are less likely to offer benefits than larger firms (Escarce and Kapur 2006). In our sample there was only a small difference in the proportion of non-Hispanic white males and Mexican-Origin males employed in very small firms, even though other researchers find major differences in the size of firms in which different racial and ethnic groups are employed (Quinn 2000). Our data are consistent with the literature in finding that Mexican-origin workers are less likely than non-Hispanic whites and blacks/African-Americans to be employed in the largest firms, which are most likely to offer benefits.

So far we have established that Mexican-origin workers are concentrated in certain occupational sectors in which their vulnerability to a lack of benefits is increased. If the lower rates of coverage among Mexican-origin male workers are to a significant extent a reflection of this concentration in certain occupations we might expect to find smaller differences within more detailed occupational categories than we have examined so far. Table 4.2 presents health insurance coverage information for the two groups of male workers within a select group of occupations. This list includes occupational categories in which the difference in health insurance

Table 4.2 Occupational differences in having own employer/union health insurance by race and Mexican origin

Occupation	(A) Non-Hispanic white	(B) Mexican origin	(B)–(A) Difference
Inspectors, testers, sorters, samplers	71.8	27.0	–44.8**
Packaging, filling machine operators	82.9	47.3	–35.6**
Electricians	68.5	34.1	–34.4**
Packers and packagers	58.9	28.0	–30.9**
Pipelayers, plumbers, pipefitters	60.5	33.2	–27.2**
Janitors and building cleaners	65.5	39.0	–26.5**
Automotive service technicians	49.3	24.4	–24.9**
Roofers	38.0	13.4	–24.5**
Production workers	77.6	53.1	–24.5**
Metal and plastic workers	86.4	62.2	–24.2**
Construction managers	54.3	51.2	–3.1
Sales representatives in services	76.2	74.9	–1.3
Butchers, meat/poultry/fish workers	59.7	59.7	0
Police and sheriff's patrol officers[a]	92.4	94.6[b,a]	+2.2
List contains this % of all employed males 18–64 years	11.1	14.8	–

* $p \leq 0.05$; ** $p \leq 0.01$.
[a]Although below the threshold ($N = 49$), we show the police and sheriff's patrol category because Mexican-origin males are slightly more likely than non-Hispanic white males to report coverage.
[b]Cell size is less than 50. All other cells contain a minimum of 50 persons.
Source: Annual Social and Economic Supplements, Current Population Survey (2004, 2006).

coverage between Mexican-origin males and non-Hispanic white males is largest, along with the police and sheriff's patrol officer category, where it is smallest. The last column of the table shows the difference in percentage terms between the two groups. Among inspectors, testers, sorters, samplers, and weighers 71.8% of non-Hispanic white workers have health insurance but only 27% of Mexican-origin workers have coverage, a difference of 44.8%. Among electricians 34.4% more non-Hispanic white workers have health insurance than Mexican-origin workers. Among pipe layers, plumbers, and pipe fitters the difference is 27.2%.

As one can see these are large differences and clearly reveal that some aspect of being of Mexican-origin places workers at a benefit disadvantage even within more refined occupational categories. Even with this greater specificity in job categories, though, major differences in the jobs included in these categories remain. Mexican-origin males may be employed in the most marginal jobs with the lowest qualification requirements and fewest benefit prospects even within the more detailed occupational groupings. The lack of difference in coverage among police and sheriff's patrol officers shows that in occupations in which coverage is universal, as it is in most governmental jobs, differences disappear. Unfortunately, as we have seen, few Hispanics are employed in such jobs. It is clear, therefore, that simple occupational concentration does not alone account for Mexican-origin benefit vulnerability. Other individual or structural characteristics contribute to their serious lack of benefits.

In order to examine the correlates of low rates of health insurance coverage among employed Mexican-origin males, we conducted several multivariate analyses that are presented elsewhere (Angel et al. 2009). Here we summarize those findings in order to provide more insight into the Mexican-origin health insurance disadvantage. In the multivariate analyses, we predicted health insurance coverage as a function of race and Mexican-origin, the occupational category, industry (i.e., manufacturing, services, construction and agriculture, professional as the reference group), work hours, employment sector (self-employed, public, private as the reference), whether the respondent had dependent coverage during the previous calendar year, and demographic characteristics, including age, education, marital status, citizenship status, and family income-to-poverty ratio.

The analyses showed that these control variables account for much of the Mexican-origin, as well as African-American, disadvantage in health insurance coverage. These multivariate analyses clearly reveal the elevated risk associated with low levels of education. They also illustrate health insurance benefits associated with marriage, including terminated marriages, older age, US citizenship, higher family income, and larger family size. The fact that Mexican-origin males have very low levels of education and are very likely not to be citizens clearly contributes to the groups' low benefit levels. These analyses show, then, that even after controlling for occupation and sector, individual-level demographic factors represent a clear health insurance risk for Mexican-origin male workers.

The Weakness of the Male Breadwinner

The available data then document serious vulnerabilities among Hispanic males, and especially among Mexican-origin males, in job-related retirement and healthcare coverage. These vulnerabilities have important implications for Hispanic families and children, as well as for the men themselves. We end with some assessment of the potential social consequences of the low human capital and limited earnings potential of such a large segment of the Hispanic male workforce. Given the centrality of the role of provider to a male's role set, a man's inability to provide adequately has serious implications, both for families and for the larger community. Males who cannot provide for all of their family's needs are deprived of a major source of satisfaction, as well as of a major source of authority and respect (Wilson 1996). They are also less able to serve as pillars of the community or to contribute to the collective economic prosperity. As we have seen, jobs without benefits are those that do not pay well and that leave a family without the economic resources to control important aspects of their lives. The employment basis of social welfare in the United States clearly places Hispanic males at a disadvantage in terms of their breadwinner role (Landale et al. 2006; Landale and Oropesa 2007). As we saw in Chapter 2, even the children of employed Hispanic parents are disproportionately dependent on Medicaid and other public programs. These children do not grow up in households in which the male parent is a socially powerful individual who can care for his family without charity or having to resort to stigmatized means-tested public programs.

Such a male cannot serve as the ideal role model for his children. Men with little education and little human capital cannot demonstrate middle-class values related to personal control and upward social mobility by example. Of course we must observe that poverty, low educational levels, and low-wage occupations are not an inevitable barrier to effective parenting or even to the possibility of upward social mobility. Many middle-class individuals grew up in very poor families in which they learned the value of education, hard work, and perseverance. Parenting takes place in a social context and has much to do with the community in which families live their lives, in addition to individual parental traits. William Julius Wilson has observed that in past decades while many neighborhoods might have been poor, they also shared the characteristic of being closely knit communities in which adult authority was clear and children could grow up in relative safety (Wilson 1987). Today that community cohesiveness is absent in many poor neighborhoods and many fathers are absent from their children's lives (Wilson, 2009). In such places effective parenting presents unique challenges, as parents must compete with gangs and with individuals who gain social status through illegal means as role models for their children. In such neighborhoods a father's inability to provide alternatives may undermine his children's chances of becoming members of the middle class.

The employment vulnerability we have documented is clearly associated with low levels of human capital. As we have shown, Hispanic males, and again especially Mexican-origin males, have extremely low levels of education. Their high school dropout rates remain shockingly high and their higher educational attainment limited, which means that a large fraction of Hispanic males simply do not qualify for good jobs. A male without a high school degree cannot pursue higher levels of education, which further limits his occupational choices. Low levels of education also increase the probability of long-term unemployment and increase the chances that a male will turn to illegal activity. With a criminal record in addition to low levels of education, the chances that a person can find any employment, and especially employment that pays well enough to provide a family with a decent living, are extremely low (Braithwaite 2005). The lack of education might lead some to blame the individual himself for his plight. If one fails to graduate from high school or if one engages in criminal activity what does one expect in terms of employment? Unfortunately, the problem is more serious than such individualistic explanations recognize; the problem is rooted in complex historical processes that result in structural barriers to educational attainment. As shown in Chapter 2, Hispanic children frequently attend inferior primary and secondary schools from which they often drop out and even when they do not, they graduate less well prepared to succeed in college than non-Hispanic white students. With mediocre college records they are less likely to pursue post-graduate education. Unlike middle-class children and adolescents, children who grow up in poor neighborhoods do see their fathers and their friends' fathers going off to well-paying jobs that give the family high social standing. Instead, young Hispanic children are three times as likely as non-Hispanic whites to have a parent in prison (Mumola 2000).

Almost in an epidemiological sense, without a critical mass of individuals with high levels of education, the community as a whole lacks the educational capital that serves as its own motivation. In order to remedy this situation, educational levels must be greatly increased among a significant number of Hispanic men and women, a proposal we return to in the final chapter.

Trapped at the Bottom

In this chapter and in previous work, we have asked the question as to the possibility that the explanation for the health insurance deficit in the Mexican-origin population reflects the concentration of Mexican-origin workers in sectors and occupations with generally low levels of coverage. The available data clearly show that Hispanic and particularly Mexican-origin males are overrepresented in low-wage jobs in which benefits are less common than they are in occupations higher in the occupational hierarchy. This concentration in low-benefit jobs certainly occurs and this fact contributes to the explanation of low rates of coverage among Mexican-origin male workers, but it is not the sole explanation. Even within sectoral and occupational categories Mexican-origin male workers have far lower rates of coverage than either non-Hispanic white or African-American male workers.

Other employment characteristics, including more part-time employment and low representation in public sector jobs contribute to low rates of coverage. These occupational factors are clearly associated with low levels of individual human capital, but they are also related to other labor markets, such as those related to the region of residence. The answer to the question as to why the Hispanic, and especially the Mexican-origin, population is at such high risk of lacking retirement plans or health insurance, then, is more complicated than a simple occupational concentration explanation would suggest. We suspect that even within the large occupational categories that are possible with CPS data, there is great variation in the quality of jobs and we suspect that within these large categories Hispanics hold those with the lowest pay and the fewest benefits. What is surprising, though, is that even at higher levels of education and income, Hispanics lag behind non-Hispanic whites in essential employment-based benefits.

Even with the large CPS sample it is impossible to examine the effects of such factors as specific job and firm size on the probability of health insurance coverage. It is likely that Mexican-origin workers, and especially the foreign-born who have low average levels of education, are employed in the smallest firms within the occupational categories we analyzed. Such small firms are less likely than large firms to offer retirement or group health insurance plans. Unfortunately we do not know from the available data whether a worker did not have the option of participating in employment-based benefit plans or whether he was offered coverage but chose not to accept it. For Mexican-origin workers with large families the premium for an employer-sponsored group health plan may simply be too high.

The risk of lacking essential benefits, then, appears to stem from multiple sources that are as yet incompletely understood and that require much more investigation. The disadvantages the Hispanic population faces probably operate interactively and at multiple levels. Hispanics, and especially the foreign-born and those who are not citizens, are less likely than non-Hispanic whites to be employed in government, education, or law enforcement in which benefit packages are almost universal. A fuller understanding of the role of structural factors on the risk of lacking benefits requires new data with richer information on firm size, the availability and cost of retirement plans and health insurance, and the employees' decision-making process concerning participation.

We end this chapter by focusing on the consequences of limited benefits for the men themselves. In our current employment-based social welfare system those at highest risk of lacking basic health coverage are adults with no disabilities. As we will document in the next chapter, the health vulnerabilities of adult women are also serious for the same reasons. For adults who are unemployed or are in jobs that do not offer health coverage, there are few options other than charity or emergency rooms. Charity and emergency rooms are hardly the most efficient and effective means of dealing with the health conditions that the poor and minorities are most likely to suffer. Policy solutions or health-care reforms that do not deal adequately with the problems of uninsured workers are likely to be ineffective in guaranteeing the optimal health of the population. Given the fact that the United States is the only developed nation without universal health-care coverage, understanding and addressing the serious vulnerabilities of Hispanics are crucial if we are to design a welfare state that addresses the needs of the most vulnerable workers and their families and that guarantees the economic future of the entire nation.

Chapter 5
Family, Work, and Benefits for Hispanic Women

In the last chapter we documented the extent of benefit disadvantage among Hispanic males and showed the particularly precarious situation of Mexican-origin men. The data make it clear that those disadvantages result from multiple sources including human capital deficits and labor market factors that confine large numbers of Hispanic male workers to low-paying jobs in construction, agriculture, and the service sector and in small firms that do not offer health or retirement benefits. In this chapter we examine the situation of adult Hispanic women and ask how their access to benefits is affected by marriage, as well as their own employment. For women, and especially for those whose culture places great value on the family and defines a woman's core roles as those of wife and mother, dependency on a male partner is common. Yet given limited earnings and the lack of benefits among Hispanic males, for many Hispanic women marriage is no guarantee of economic security or access to health insurance or retirement income. As is the case for lower class African-American women, for a large fraction of Hispanic women the traditional male-breadwinner model of family economic security no longer operates, if indeed it ever did, and the future marriage market for Hispanic females may operate very differently than it has in the past. For women in general, their unique economic vulnerabilities can be traced in large part to the fact that the employment-based benefit system that emerged after World War II in the United States was firmly based on the male-breadwinner model of family economic security. That model, which was historically precarious for lower class woman, has become increasingly unreliable in assuring a family's economic security.

In the idealized traditional family the male partner's role is to serve as the primary or sole breadwinner while his wife remains home to manage the house and raise the children (Moen and Roehling 2004). Although the reality of family life has changed profoundly and the number of single-parent households has increased among all racial and ethnic groups, the male-breadwinner model continues to form the basis of many social welfare policies as well as public expectations. The two-parent family is still the ideal in the public mind, and for traditionalists it remains the optimal if not the only environment in which to successfully raise children. The fact that a single parent must often assume the full financial burden of the household without anyone to share domestic and childrearing tasks gives some credence to this value judgment. There can be little doubt that the earnings disadvantage faced by single women

R.J. Angel, J.L. Angel, *Hispanic Families at Risk*, DOI 10.1007/978-1-4419-0474-4_5,

greatly increases the potential stressors associated with single motherhood. Despite the desire to preserve the traditional two-parent family, though, demographic and social realities have changed and are unlikely to return to what they were.

Today women enter the labor force at rates almost as high as those of men and younger women are as career oriented as their male peers. Increasingly, women do not expect marriage to assure their own or their children's economic well-being. As the new social reality of marriage and family takes hold, women must face the fact that an adult female's role set includes that of worker in addition to that of parent. Women who do not work or those who exit and reenter the labor force in response to family needs lose both earnings and benefits, as well as the continuity and potential mobility of a career. Women are simply finding that by choice or necessity they need to work. Yet as is the case for men, the economic rewards of work can be limited. Those rewards depend on many individual and job-related factors as well as on gender-based labor force factors that result in lower earnings for women than for men. In 2002 non-Hispanic white women earned on average 78.2% of what non-Hispanic men earned. Perhaps because of the more limited earnings capacities of minority men, in that same year African-American women earned 90.2% of what African-American men earned and Hispanic women earned 88.2% of what Hispanic men earned (Bureau of Labor Statistics 2003). Women, therefore, face many of the same challenges as men to economic security through work, with the added disadvantage of a gender-based wage penalty. As we will show, this gender-based penalty interacts with a minority penalty to place Hispanic women in a particularly disadvantaged position.

The ethnicity penalty is revealed by the fact that the earnings of employed Mexican-origin women are considerably lower than those of non-Hispanic white and African-American women. In 2000 African-American women earned 95% of what non-Hispanic white women earned but Mexican-origin women earned only 60% as much (Duncan et al. 2006). These low earnings among Hispanic women are largely accounted for by the foreign-born; while native-born women earn 84% of what non-Hispanic white women earn, foreign-born women earn only 37% as much. There can be little doubt, then, that gender, minority group status, and nativity each represent important dimensions of disadvantage, and in combination they clearly define the most vulnerable individuals in our society. Although an upper middle class non-Hispanic white professional woman may experience gender-based disadvantages in terms of promotion and income, she is in a very different situation than a foreign-born Hispanic domestic worker who works for minimum wage if she is lucky. If one adds single motherhood to this pool of factors, the result is an even more precarious economic profile and one in which a large fraction of children, and especially minority children, find themselves today. In 2007, 58% of African-American, 28% of Hispanic children, and 19% of non-Hispanic children were growing up in a female-headed household (U.S. Census Bureau 2008b). For single women with children, work or welfare or both are the only options for even minimal economic security. Unfortunately, given the labor force disadvantages that women with little education face, work is often a dead end. For African-American women the average level of education is 12.9 years and for non-Hispanic white women it is 13.7 years (Everett et al. 2007). The average educational attainment of Mexican-origin women is less than high school among the native-born and just 9 years for the foreign-born. For many of the foreign-born, the little education they have was often obtained in Mexico and may have been of low quality.

Nonetheless, because they are often the sole providers for their families, African-American women have historically worked and they have had more continuous labor force attachment than non-Hispanic white women (Yoon 1996). Unlike professionals, poor women who take marginal jobs do not work for self-fulfillment or satisfaction, they do so of necessity. Many Mexican-origin women work out of financial necessity because the low earnings of Mexican-origin men are inadequate to support large families, even if the supposed cultural norm for Hispanic women is that of homemaker (Moreno and Muller 1996). For minority women, work and family life are interconnected in new and evolving ways that reflect a new social reality.

The social reality of marriage and family is changing in ways that do not bode well for the traditional family form, even among Hispanics. Although the traditional family form lies at the core of many people's conception of an orderly society the cultural, economic, and social forces that supported the traditional family in specific cultural and historical contexts are under extreme stress in our modern globalized world. In traditional peasant societies, such as those characteristic of Mexican villages in the not too distant past, marriage was a cultural imperative and large families was the norm to which one had no choice but to conform. In such societies men provided a minimal level of economic support through basic agrarian and other subsistence activities. The stability and stasis of such a cultural arrangement have been torn asunder by rural to urban and international migration. In the urban environment and in more modern societies, a man's ability to provide materially takes on a new meaning. To provide for his family a male must negotiate the urban labor market, a task that is very difficult if one has little education and is not fluent in the language. In order to thrive in urban Mexico or in the United States, basic peasant-level skills or productivity are not enough, and true economic security requires more education, skills, and the ability to deal with complex social organizations. As time passes, and as Hispanic families adopt the norms of the new urban environment, women may find that the men whom they might have married as the result of social convention are no longer desirable since they cannot provide economic security.

Yet even as gender roles change and as the traditional family declines, our basic vision of the economic role of marriage has only recently begun to adjust to this new reality. In the traditional view of marriage a woman marries early in life and remains married to the same male until one member of the couple dies. During her childrearing years a wife depends on her husband's income and family health insurance policy for economic security and health care. After age 65 she enjoys the security that the couple's accumulated assets and her husband's retirement plans provide. Although she may have worked temporarily, the primary source of her income, her health-care coverage, and her retirement security are her husband's employment. In the traditional view, family and not work define a woman's role set.

This idealized life course based on early and continuous marriage to a single partner is increasingly irrelevant for large segments of the female population. Indeed, for many women married to men with low earnings capacities, including a large fraction of Hispanic and African-American women, marriage never has provided financial security. Today the increase in the number of women who cannot depend on marriage for financial security is growing. This growth comes from several sources with which most of us are familiar. A growing number of women never marry or have children; others never marry the fathers of the children they do have; yet others divorce, often more than once. Even when they do marry, though, for many women marriage provides little real economic security or access to benefits. A husband with high earnings and good benefits may provide his wife a comfortable and secure life; a husband with a low earnings capacity and no benefits cannot provide that same comfort or security. Let us examine some of the demographic and social changes in family and work that affect Hispanic and other minority women in today's world.

The Decline of the Family

The changing nature of the family represents a cultural shift of monumental proportions and is the reason why we devote a separate chapter to women's access to benefits. In earlier times we might well have approached the issue of benefit coverage as a family matter and examined only the male breadwinner's access to health insurance and retirement coverage. Such an approach is no longer reasonable since many women find themselves responsible for their own and their family's economic security and access to health care. The fact that women are responsible for children and the home makes the analysis of their employment behavior and access to benefits more complicated than is the case for men. Changing marital and family realities mean that a woman's source of income and social benefits can change with her marital status and her own employment, potentially several times during her lifetime. Understanding women's economic situation generally, then, requires the simultaneous examination of her family and work roles.

Although increasing rates of marital disruption are a major cause of increased female employment, women's entry into the labor market has also been fueled by a general increase in consumption levels (Coontz 2000). Owning a home, two cars, and all of the material accessories that have come to define a middle-class American lifestyle increasingly requires two incomes. For lower class women and their families simply making do often represents a daunting challenge. Although many women work simply to supplement household income, a growing number do not see their work as only temporary or supplemental. This commitment to a career is reflected in the dramatic increase in the number of women who earn professional degrees. Between 1979–1980 and 2005–2006 the number of women doubled earning professional degrees, from 3,486 to 7,555 in law and 7,555 to 20,843 in medicine (National Center for Education Statistics 2007a). Today, more than half of students admitted to law schools and medical schools are women and women are taking their places in government, academia, and business (National Center for Education Statistics 2007a). Women are also assuming a greater responsibility for their own retirement and health benefits. Yet for many women, and especially minority women, work is no guarantee of an adequate income or benefits. While highly educated professional women have access to retirement and health plans, poorly educated women who work in the low-wage service sector usually do not. Despite the growing number of women with their own benefit coverage, marriage continues to represent a major source of economic well-being and access to health benefits for a large fraction of women (Moen and Roehling 2004; Meyer and Herd 2007). Women with little education and no specialized skills have limited employment opportunities. In addition, institutionalized gender role expectations place women at a disadvantage relative to men in terms of access to benefits and increase their reliance on a male breadwinner (Pascall and Lewis 2004; Orloff 1993). Unfortunately, for minority women that breadwinner is very often limited in what he can provide.

The changing demographic and social reality that is rapidly transforming marriage and family life has especially significant implications for minority women, including Hispanic women. Minority status interacts with gender to place Hispanic and African-American women at elevated risk of economic insecurity throughout life. Although one might argue that minority group status trumps gender as a dimension of disadvantage or vice versa, there can be no doubt that together, gender, race, and Hispanic ethnicity form the major dimensions of labor market segmentation and economic vulnerability in the United States today. The cumulative disadvantage that the combination of minority group status and female gender entails has serious negative consequences not only for a woman's economic well-being but also for her physical and mental health as well as that of her children. An inadequate income and a lack of health insurance not only increase health risks but undermine a woman's ability to obtain care for herself and her family. This serious interactive impact of gender and minority status on women's and children's well-being is rooted in a long history of minority exclusion in the United States as well as institutionalized gender-based economic disadvantages that interact with race and Hispanic ethnicity to undermine access to health care and retirement security for minority women.

As we did for men in the last chapter, we pay particular attention to the labor force situation of Mexican-origin women. Our justification for focusing on Mexican-origin women is the same as it was for focusing on Mexican-origin men; at all ages the Mexican-origin population has by far the highest level of income insecurity and the lowest rate of benefit coverage of any racial or ethnic group in the United States (Escarce and Kapur 2006). In addition, cultural norms associated with familism and masculine dominance that are often held to be characteristic of Mexican culture may exaggerate gender-based differences and further weaken the occupational options of Mexican-origin women (see Vandello and Cohen 2003). The core question we address, then, is whether Hispanic women's marital and family statuses influence their employment experiences, and ultimately their health insurance coverage and retirement security.

Gender, Hispanic Ethnicity, and Access to Benefits

Since they are for the most part employment benefits, access to retirement plans and health insurance depends upon the quality of one's job. Almost by definition, a good job is one that provides not only a good salary but also benefits. Access to adequate health care and a secure retirement, then, depends on possessing the human capital that qualifies one for a good job and a career. Given the important role of marriage in securing benefits for women, access to benefits depends on a husband's human capital as well as that of his wife. As we saw in the last chapter, for Hispanics as a whole and Mexican-origin families in particular, low levels of human capital are a major barrier to adequate benefits. Low levels of human capital limit the type of jobs for which many Hispanics qualify. Minority women face an elevated risk of inadequate benefit coverage for several reasons, including their own often limited human capital. As we will see, Mexican-origin women are disproportionately confined to low-wage occupations that do not offer coverage and they are more likely than non-Hispanic white women to be married to men who do not have benefit coverage.

Figure 5.1 shows that among women aged 25–64 years African-Americans are the most likely to be employed with 78% in the civilian labor force, followed closely by non-Hispanic white women at 71.4%, native-born Mexican-origin women at 68.4%, and finally, foreign-born Mexican-origin women at 45.2%. Again reflecting their more traditional domestic roles, employment rates are far lower among foreign-born Mexican-origin women than among the native-born; while 68.4% of native-born women are in the labor force, only 45.2% of foreign-born women are employed.

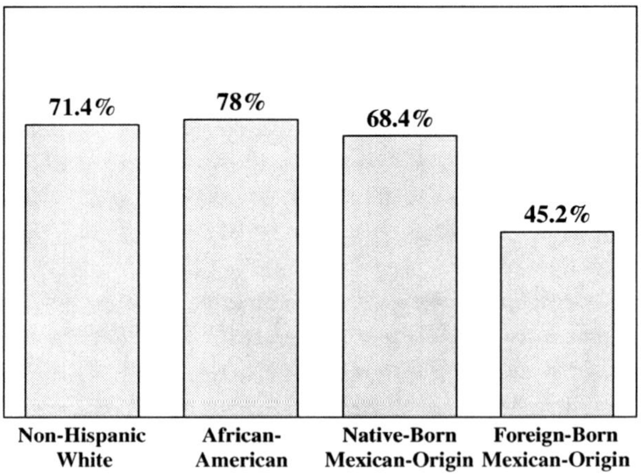

Figure 5.1 Employed women aged 25–64 years by race, Mexican ethnicity, and nativity, 2006
Source: Current Population Survey (2004, 2006).

The more traditional orientation of Mexican-origin women is revealed in Fig. 5.2, which shows that Mexican-origin women are especially likely to stay at home to raise children. As a result of higher fertility, Hispanic women put in fewer years at work and lose out on years of paying into a retirement plan (Landale and Oropesa 2007). Fertility cannot wait and occurs during the prime working years, resulting in

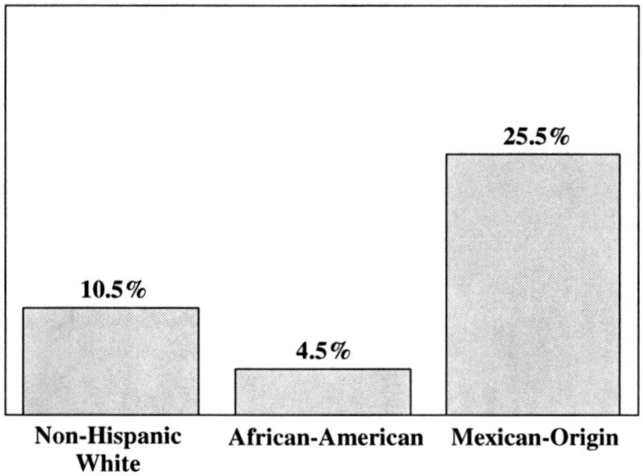

Figure 5.2 Stay-at-home mothers by race, Mexican ethnicity, and nativity, 2006 *Source:* Current Population Survey (2004–2006).

an inevitable tradeoff between having children and working. The types of work that women with little education qualify for do not offer the maternity leaves that professional women can often rely upon. Women who choose to take time out to raise children, or who are forced to do so by necessity, lose those prime working years and when they return to the workforce they do so at the same level at which they left, often with obsolete skills, giving them even less opportunity to save. Given the limited work opportunities available to many of these women, their own employment is unlikely to compensate for the economic weakness of marriage. Few of the service sector jobs for which they qualify are likely to provide even minimal benefit packages that include a retirement plan. These sources of vulnerability in conjunction with the increasing longevity among the Mexican-origin population may result in women outliving their savings or the meager assets they and their spouse were able to accumulate.

Figure 5.3 shows, compared with non-Hispanic white and African-American women, Hispanic women are overrepresented in benefit-poor service occupations. In 2008, they are also less likely than African-American and non-Hispanic white working women to belong to unions (10% versus 13.3 and 11.1%, respectively) (Bureau of Labor Statistics 2009c). Because undocumented Mexican women have limited opportunities to work in the formal sector, most find informal employment in which benefits do not exist (Hondagneu-Sotelo 1997). Even when they work Hispanic women, and especially Mexican-origin women, are less likely than non-Hispanic women to work in occupations that offer benefits. Given their low levels of education, it is not surprising that Mexican-origin women are far less likely than non-Hispanic white women and even African-American women to be employed in management and professional occupations (Santos and Seitz 2000).

This economic and benefit disadvantage among Hispanics begins early in life and continues into old age. As we showed earlier, Mexican-origin individuals are the least likely of any racial or ethnic group to have health insurance at all ages. Mexican-origin children are far less likely to be insured than non-Hispanic white,

Figure 5.3
Professional/Service Sector Employment by Race/Ethnicity
Source: Current Population Survey, 2008.

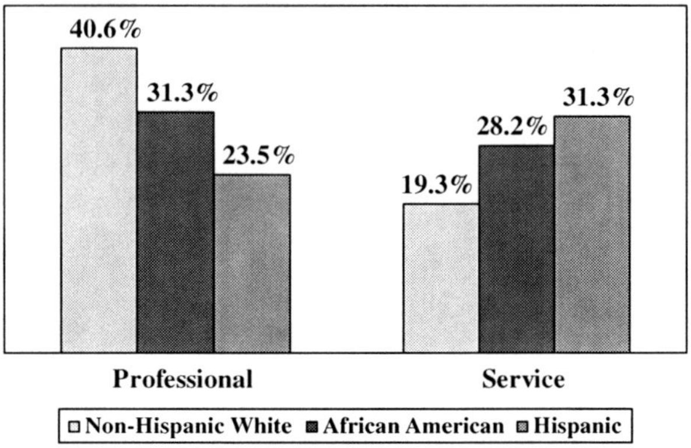

African-American, or other Hispanic children (Angel et al. 2007; Hamilton et al. 2006). Forty-five percent of Mexican-origin adults have no health insurance, compared with 25% of Cuban-Americans, 23% of Puerto Ricans, 24% of African-Americans, and 13% of non-Hispanic whites (Angel et al. 2007). Mexican-origin families are far more likely than other families to have incomplete family coverage, a situation in which some members are covered but others are not (Angel et al. 2007; Amey et al. 1995). In the years prior to retirement, older Mexican-origin adults continue to have lower rates of coverage than other groups and after retirement they are less likely to have supplemental Medigap health insurance to cover the costs that Medicare does not pay (Angel and Angel 1996). The situation is especially problematic for married women with husbands who are eligible for Medicare and for older Mexican-origin women in particular (Angel et al. 2009).

Marriage as a Source of Benefit Coverage

Given the fact that marriage continues to be one of the primary sources of benefit coverage for women and their children, we must examine the marriage/benefits connection in some detail. For many women marriage is still a source of coverage (Montez et al. 2009). Married women are more likely to have private health insurance than divorced or never married women and they are less likely than unmarried women to rely on publicly funded sources for health care for their children (Anderson and Eamon 2004; Bernstein et al. 2008; Meyer and Pavalko 1996; Hahn 1993). Married women also have more continuous coverage than single women (Short 1998).

Of course the likelihood of having coverage through marriage is conditioned by the likelihood of getting married. For women the likelihood of marriage depends on the availability of marriageable males. For minority women the pool of marriageable males, meaning those with good earnings and benefit prospects, can be rather small (Wilson 1987). The lack of marriageable males is particularly serious for African-American women who are less likely to be married than either non-Hispanic white or Mexican-origin women (U.S. Census Bureau 2006a). Although Hispanic women still marry at high rates the changing nature of modern labor markets, as well as changing cultural expectations, may reduce the marriage rate in the future. As we mentioned in the introduction to this chapter, in traditional cultures a woman marries and remains married to a man because of societal norms and men's occupational qualifications remain limited to those necessary for agrarian tasks. These motivations to marry may weaken in the United States as the earnings capacities of poorly educated Hispanic males become more of a problem. When norms cease to force women to marry men with little earnings potential, the forces that work against marriage will, in all likelihood, become more salient.

Recent studies indicate that while marriage provides economic security, including health-care security, to middle-class non-Hispanic white women, it does not necessarily do so for minority and poor women. In fact, the evidence suggests that while non-Hispanic white women tend to benefit economically from marriage, African-American women benefit more from their own employment (Angel et al. 2007; Lupton and Smith 2003; Willson 2003). Other evidence for the selective benefits of marriage is provided by the fact that while for non-Hispanic white women marriage increases the odds of having a family income above poverty, it does not necessarily do the same for Hispanic women (Lichter et al. 2003).

Several factors help to explain the more-limited economic benefits of marriage for Hispanic women. Hispanic women tend to marry at earlier ages than non-Hispanic women, a factor associated with both low educational levels and an elevated risk of poverty (Oropesa et al. 1994). Hispanic, and especially Mexican-origin, fertility rates are higher than those of the population at large (Oropesa 1996). Hispanics begin having children at earlier ages than other groups, which is also associated with lower educational levels. In one study, Hispanic middle school girls, most of whom were Mexican-origin, reported lower educational and job aspirations and a greater desire to marry and become mothers than non-Hispanic white or African-American girls (East 1998). These lower educational aspirations have serious consequences. While demographers usually treat education as a predictor of fertility, the opposite holds as well. Girls who become pregnant early often drop out of school and marry partners with little education and few job opportunities. Early marriage, low educational levels, and limited occupational opportunities, then, undermine mobility chances for individuals and families, especially among Mexican immigrants (Landale and Oropesa 2007; Raley et al. 2004).

The timing of motherhood has profound consequences for a woman's economic and occupational life course trajectory (Moen and Roehling 2004; Spain and Bianchi 1996). Women remain primarily responsible for children, and as a consequence employed women are more likely to reduce work hours or temporarily exit the labor force in response to family demands than are employed men. It comes as no surprise then that motherhood is associated with lower wages and fewer fringe benefits, an effect of parenthood that is opposite to that for men (Moen and Roehling 2004). Partly as a result of the inherent conflict between employment and family demands, many middle-class women have responded by delaying or foregoing marriage and childbearing (Spain and Bianchi 1996). For marriage to serve as a life-long source of health and retirement benefits, it must not only be to a male with work-related benefits but also be continuous and a woman must be married without significant interruption (Wood et al. 2007). Given the growing reality of marital instability, access to spousal benefits can end abruptly. If a woman does not remarry, marriage ceases to serve as a source of benefits. If one is married for less than 10 years one cannot claim a portion of a previous spouse's Social Security. A woman's current marital status, then, rather than her marital history, is the significant predictor of her benefit status (Meyer and Pavalko 1996). As a consequence, for women reliance on marriage alone as a source of benefit coverage, as well as for economic well-being generally, is increasingly risky (Wood et al. 2007). Married women who have health insurance as dependents are more likely than those who have their own coverage to lose that insurance over time (Short 1998).

Employment as a Source of Benefit Coverage

Although marriage continues to be a major source of economic security and health insurance for women, employment is rapidly assuming an equally important role. The simple reality of modern life is that, like it or not, women are forced to deal with economic issues that in the past they left to their husbands (Bernstein et al. 2008). Yet even as employment becomes the norm for women, as is the case for men, race and ethnicity structure employment opportunities unequally, a situation that results in unequal access to material and social resources including retirement plans and health insurance (Heinz 2004; Misra 1999; Higginbotham 1997). The differential access to health insurance and other benefits among women is influenced by several factors, including their level of education, their employment statuses, the nature of the jobs they hold, and the number of hours they works, as well as the labor market opportunities in the region, state, and locality in which they live.

For workers and their families the continuity of employment benefits and health insurance is of major importance. One of the major shortcomings of public programs is that the care they provide is often discontinuous, incomplete, and temporary. Poor families often experience periods during which some of the children in the family have no health coverage while others receive Medicaid (Angel et al. 2006). Retirement plans and health insurance are largely restricted to individuals who maintain continuous full-time employment (Moen and Roehling 2004; Heinz 2004). Long periods of unemployment, part-time work, or episodic employment that reflect low levels of human capital undermine retirement planning and savings generally.

Work and Retirement Security

Negative life events or chronic hardships, including widowhood, divorce, job layoffs, one's own or a family member's health problems, or disability can drain a woman's resources and make it impossible for her to devote time to work. Combined with inadequate savings and incomplete retirement preparations, the financial impact can be devastating. Certain evidence suggests that these forms of financial risks are greatest for older minority group women (Hounsell et al. 2006). Our own analysis of women's retirement coverage based on the CPS corroborates these findings; older Mexican-origin women experience more of these adverse life events than other groups. The financial vulnerability faced by the female Mexican-origin population also reflects other factors, which in and of themselves represent positive demographic trends. During the 20th century life expectancy at birth and at older ages increased for all racial and ethnic groups (Angel and Hogan 2004). At age 65 years Mexican-origin women have a life expectancy similar to if not higher than that of non-Hispanic white women (Eschbach et al. 2007). At the age of 65 years, Hispanic women can expect to live an additional 22.8 years, 2.9 years longer than non-Hispanic White women and 4.2 years longer than African-American women (Center for American Progress 2004). As their life expectancies increase, older Hispanic women are likely to outlive their husbands, at the same time that they suffer the chronic and disabling illnesses that accompany aging. Many of these women will outlive their resources and find themselves dependent on children or the state.

Figure 5.4 presents data from the 2006 CPS comparing the extent of retirement coverage among working-age Mexican-origin and non-Hispanic women between the ages of 25 and 64 years. In the CPS, 41.7% of Mexican-origin adult women report that they are covered by a retirement plan from some source. Fifty-eight percent of African-American women and 61.4% of non-Hispanic white women report such coverage. Unfortunately, the CPS does not provide information on the type or source of retirement plan a woman has or whether she has coverage on her own (Sanzenbacher 2006). Among those women 50 years and older who own a retirement plan, the median annual benefit in 2007 was only 64.6% of that received by men, $13,573 compared with $19,787 (Employee Benefit Research Institute 2008). Although we do not have information by racial and ethnic group, we suspect that the amount of retirement income received by Mexican-origin women is less than that

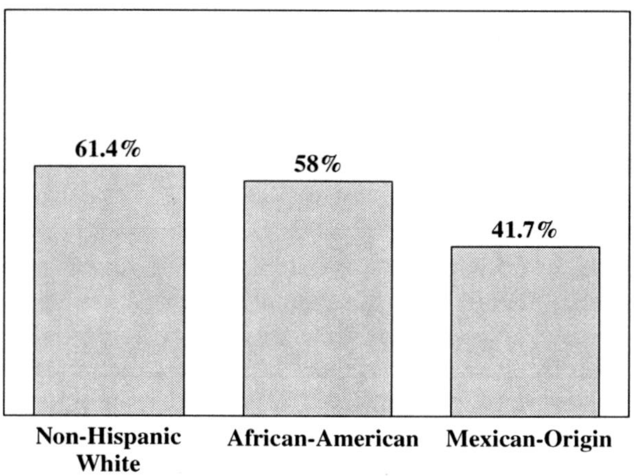

Figure 5.4 Any pension coverage for women aged 25–64 years, 2006
Source: Current Population Survey (2004, 2006).

received by non-Hispanic white women for two reasons related to the labor market disadvantages we have already noted; Mexican-origin women have historically had lower wages and earnings than non-Hispanic white women and they marry men who do not have benefits.

Once again, low levels of education are a major source of the problem, Hispanic women, and especially those of Mexican origin, have very low levels of education, which limits their career choices and keeps their incomes low. Mexican-origin workers have the lowest educational levels among Hispanics. Their returns to education are lower than for other groups, and especially for the foreign-born since US employers tend to place less value on education obtained in Mexico (Thomas et al. 2006). Without an education, occupational mobility is unlikely and many Hispanic women move from one low-wage hourly job to the next with no increase in job-related human capital. Without the ability to acquire valuable skills one has little to offer but physical labor. In addition, as we have noted before, Hispanics contribute less to their 401(k)s even when they own them, a fact exacerbated by the youth of the Mexican-origin population since younger workers tend to contribute less to retirement plans than older workers (Orszag and Rodriguez 2005).

Social Security

As a result of the low levels of private retirement coverage Social Security takes on a major role in providing income support in old age for Hispanics. More than half of the total income of Hispanic couples 65 years or older comes from Social Security compared with 45.6% among non-Hispanic white couples (Social Security Administration 2000). Again revealing the unique vulnerability of the foreign born, women who were born in Mexico are the least likely of any group to participate in the Social Security program and they are at the highest risk of poverty in old age (Ham-Chande 2008; Hendley and Bilimoria 1999). Foreign-born women are less likely than native-born women to have contributed the required 10 years themselves and they are often married to men who also did not make the required contribution, leaving their wives ineligible for the surviving spouse's portion of Social Security. Some have suggested that women born in Mexico are not prepared for work in the United States (Ham-Chande 2008). Immigrant women face multiple employment barriers including low educational levels, low levels of English proficiency, and the lack of legal documentation (Hondagneu-Sotelo 2001). If they find work as domestics or in the informal economy, their employers often do not contribute to Social Security in their names (Baker 1999).

As we mentioned in the last chapter, but reiterate here because of its importance in understanding the situation of Hispanics and of Hispanic women in particular, Social Security was never meant to be an older person's sole source of income. Although the average woman gains relatively more than the average male from Social Security because the benefit structure favors dependents and low-wage earners, most of whom are women or children, as we showed in the last chapter average benefit levels are modest at best. Social Security was intended to be only one pillar of the theoretical three-pillared retirement arrangement, which also includes private retirement plans and individual savings. The fact that Hispanics, and especially single Hispanic females, have relatively few assets and no retirement plan increases their dependence on Social Security and means that it is frequently their only source of income and increases their risk of poverty in old age (Sevak et al. 2003–2004).

Health Insurance

In addition to retirement and social security, health-care coverage rates among Hispanic women reveal an added dimension of vulnerability. Figure 5.5 presents data from the 2006 CPS that highlights the large racial and ethnic disparities in health-care coverage among women. Overall, Mexican-origin adult women are far less likely to have coverage than non-Hispanic white. These low levels of coverage persist throughout the working years and clearly negatively affect access to high-quality and continuous health care. As the data in Fig. 5.6 show, Mexican-origin women have particularly low levels of coverage at all ages. It is not until the age of 65 years when, as we will demonstrate in Chapter 7 in which we deal with the elderly, Medicare greatly reduces this health insurance gap. Even then though, as we will see, Hispanics face continuing disadvantages in terms of complete coverage.

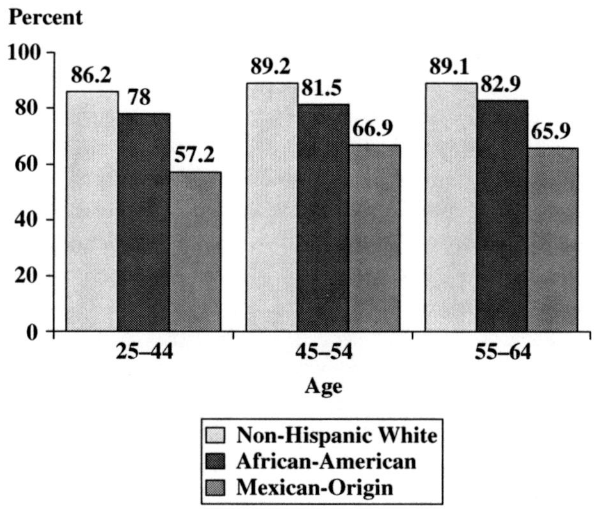

Figure 5.5 Percentage of women with any health insurance by age, 2006
Source: Current Population Survey (2004, 2006).

Mother, Worker, and Still No Benefits

We end the chapter by summarizing some of our previous multivariate analyses of the interactive impact of marriage, motherhood, and employment on the likelihood of health insurance coverage for Mexican-origin women and by speculating on how the socioeconomic vulnerabilities of Hispanic women might be addressed. We do

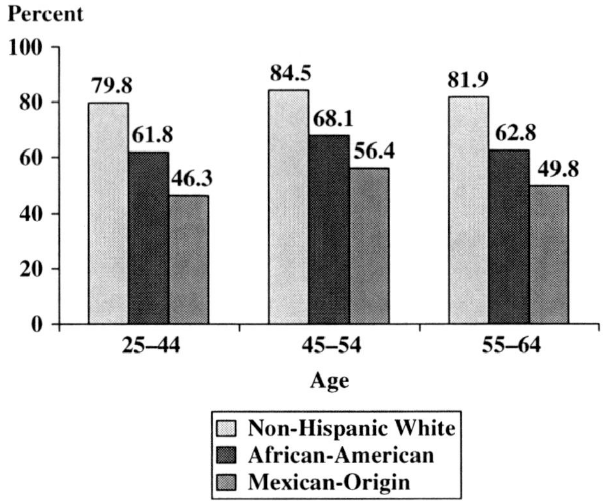

Figure 5.6 Percentage of women with private coverage by age, 2006
Source: Current Population Survey (2004, 2006).

not present the multivariate analyses here because of their complexity; rather we refer the reader to the relevant published articles (Angel et al. 2009; Montez et al. 2009). Although we will deal with policy related to the benefit poverty among Hispanics generally in the final chapter, the unique situation of women, and especially working-age women, presents serious challenges that deserve discussion in their own right. We focus on health insurance because of its importance to an individual's and a family's health and because it is a core work-related benefit. Health insurance coverage and other benefits are usually part of the same employment-based package; jobs that do not offer health insurance are likely not to offer retirement plans. Given the disparities in health coverage we have documented in this chapter, two important questions related to the interaction of work and family for women emerge. These we pose as problems for future research and as vitally important policy questions.

The core question we ask and propose for further research is whether the health insurance disparities we have documented among Mexican-origin, non-Hispanic white, and African-American women result from distinct combinations of employment and family structure that operate differently for each group. Logically this involves determining whether disparities in coverage disappear or at least diminish once we statistically control for such factors as marital status and history, fertility behavior, educational levels, employment characteristics, and nativity status among others. The ethnic and racial patterns of family and work that we have presented in this chapter suggest that combining work and family has different effects on the probability of benefit coverage because of the different jobs that various groups of women qualify for, their differential fertility and marital experiences, and factors related to culture. As we have suggested, it is unlikely that race or ethnicity alone, or gender alone, places certain women at elevated risk of low income and limited or no benefits. Rather, it is increasingly clear that different combinations of factors operate differently for each group and that for Hispanic women, and for foreign-born Mexican-origin women in particular, labor force difficulties, family demands, culture, and job opportunities interact negatively to decrease coverage. Addressing these complex interactive problems present policy makers and the Hispanic community with a great challenge.

There can be little doubt of course that low levels of education are a major source of these problems. Yet one cannot treat low levels of education as exogenous, to use the statistical term. Educational levels are part of the process by which certain groups, in this case the Mexican-origin population, are relegated to the lower social strata where their ability to move ahead is seriously compromised. Treating education as a purely individual characteristic ignores those factors, such as inferior schools and the lack of role models that we discussed in Chapter 2, that structure and institutionalize group-specific disadvantages.

These multivariate analyses we summarize here are based on the Annual Social and Economic (ASEC) Supplement to the March CPS that we have used in this and previous chapters. The sample on which they are based consists of 81,822 non-Hispanic white, African-American, and Mexican-origin women between 18 and 64 years of age who were either employed full-time or not employed. The analysis is informed by two specific theories concerning the potentially interactive roles of marriage and work in determining the likelihood of having health insurance coverage. The first is a role substitution theory, which hypothesizes that employment and marriage are substitutes for one another in providing access to health insurance (Waldron et al. 1996). The second is a role accumulation theory, which hypothesizes that the combination of marriage and employment increases the probability of coverage beyond that of marriage or employment alone (Waldron et al. 1998). The intriguing possibility, of course, is that because of group-specific historical and structural factors, marriage and work may produce different outcomes for different groups of women. As often happens in the analysis of phenomena with multiple causes, our findings support aspects of both theoretical perspectives.

What our data reveal is that after controlling for factors known to be associated with the probability of having health insurance including age, education, nativity, family income, and self-rated health, employment and marriage substitute for one another and either insures adequate health insurance coverage for non-Hispanic white women. The health insurance benefits of marriage and work are different, though, for African-American and Mexican-origin women. Employment largely compensates for lower access to spousal coverage among African-American women, but it does not for Mexican-origin women. This means that employed African-American women are more likely to have coverage regardless of their marital status than unemployed African-American women, revealing a clear employment advantage. For Mexican-origin women neither marriage nor work assures health-care coverage. The extremely low rates of health insurance coverage we have documented for the Mexican-origin population at all ages apparently result from factors other than the traditional predictors of health insurance coverage. The data also underline the extreme vulnerability of stay-at-home Mexican-origin mothers who are at the highest risk of lacking health insurance. For these women the odds of having coverage only marginally improve with employment.

The data show then that while marital and work roles substitute for each other in terms of access to health-care coverage among non-Hispanic white women, this is not the case for Mexican-origin women. Nor does it appear that work pays off in terms of coverage for Mexican-origin women in the same way it does for African-American women. Whether they are married, employed, or both, Mexican-origin women are less likely than either non-Hispanic white or African-American women to have health insurance. Mexican-origin men are evidently unable to provide their spouses and families with this vitally important work-related benefit. Given the serious educational deficits of Mexican-origin men, this situation is unlikely to change without serious attempts to increase levels of education for both Mexican-origin men and women.

The Rise of the Female Breadwinner

This research provides new insights into the sources of structural disadvantage in benefit coverage among working-age Mexican-origin women. In order to improve our understanding of the unique vulnerabilities of Hispanic women in the United States, and especially among Mexican-origin women, we must look beyond individual characteristics to the institutional factors that structure family roles and labor market opportunities. As we have noted, in the very near future Hispanics will make up a large fraction of the labor force. A large fraction of that Hispanic labor force will be female. This growth in female Hispanic labor force representation reflects three core social and cultural factors, namely high fertility, immigration, and the likely greater propensity of Hispanic women to enter the labor force. This greater labor force involvement results from, and will probably accelerate, basic changes in Hispanic family structure. For all racial and ethnic groups, the dramatic retreat from marriage and fertility that we have witnessed in recent years, accompanied by the increase in paid employment that we have documented even among Hispanic women, may dramatically alter their sources of basic social welfare benefits.

As we noted at the beginning of the chapter, the institutionalized breadwinner model of family welfare informs much public policy in the United States. Social Security, private retirement and health plans, and other benefits are tied to a male spouse's employment (Herd 2005). Even today, public expectations and employer prejudices place women, or at least lower class women, at a clear labor force disadvantage. As we noted, women make less than men and Hispanic women earn less than non-Hispanic white women. The combination of gender, minority status, and the institutionalized structures of the male-breadwinner orientation poses serious barriers to change. As the family declines even among Hispanics, women remain responsible for children and the employment possibilities of poorly educated women with little work experience are limited not only by little human capital but also by domestic responsibilities. For a single woman the combination of financial responsibility for a family and the responsibilities of parenthood can be daunting, especially when one has no choice but to raise one's children in unsafe and crime- and gang-ridden neighborhoods.

Of course it is impossible to deny that low educational attainment and a lack of English proficiency lie at the core of the problem of low-wage employment and the lack of benefits for both Hispanic men and women (Thomas et al. 2006). Addressing the problem, then, means identifying those social and institutional factors that undermine educational success for such a large fraction of the Mexican-origin population. As we have suggested earlier and will reiterate in the last chapter, until a critical mass of Hispanics achieve high levels of education and professional status, the collective economic and political power of the group as a whole will remain low. Jobs that pay well are the ones that offer retirement and health plans, but they also require higher levels of education and the sort of work-related skills that more education allows one to learn on the job and that enhance one's employability further. Cleaning motel rooms does not result in increments to one's human capital and such jobs are not part of a career ladder. In such jobs one can work for the same minimal wage for years. For these reasons, education must become the focus of attempts to improve the lot of Hispanics in general and Hispanic women in particular.

The evidence we have presented leads us to the conclusion that the male-breadwinner model of retirement security should be reconsidered, especially for minority women. Regardless of their race or ethnicity or even their social class, future cohorts of working-age women will be forced to take greater responsibility for their own welfare and retirement incomes. This will clearly require much more attention to education and enhanced human capital. Until their situation in the labor force improves, Hispanic women will remain on the lowest rungs of the occupational ladder and their children will suffer the consequences. Today middle-class women are as concerned with issues related to their careers and their financial security as are men. Even as they face restricted employment and earnings possibilities, Hispanic women will be forced to deal with financial issues as well. Because of the labor force disadvantages they face, though, the situation of low-wage service sector workers and the unemployed and underemployed requires special attention. Public policy related to health care, family welfare, and retirement income must guarantee the health and productivity of future generations of workers. For many Hispanic women employment will never serve as a route out of poverty or ensure an adequate retirement income.

For this reason, any changes to the present Social Security system will have to take these vulnerabilities into account. The long-term fiscal health of the Social Security system will require some retrenchment, including higher payroll taxes and reduced benefits. Proposals aimed at cutting benefits as opposed to generating revenue would have particularly serious implications for poor and minority women. For better or worse, the situation of these women argues for greater means testing of benefits. Such a move, of course, runs the risk of transforming Social Security into more of a welfare program with the potential stigma that welfare entails. In addition to the inevitable reforms to Social Security that we will see in the future, efforts to improve access to private pensions and increased personal savings and investment by low-wage employees of both sexes are clearly warranted, even if the possibilities remain limited (Herd 2005; Meyer and Herd 2008). The partial privatization of Social Security has been offered as a means of increasing individual returns and responsibilities. Unfortunately, such reforms would in all likelihood not improve the old-age security of low-wage workers or those with noncontinuous work histories. The privatization of Social Security without other reforms to ensure an adequate income to those without adequate savings would only increase the risk for minority paid workers.

We end with the observation that reforms to the private retirement system, to Social Security, and to the health-care financing system of the United States to insure adequate coverage for the most vulnerable citizens clearly face serious practical barriers that have been made only worse by the global economic crisis. Such challenges are inevitable and require a far better understanding of the specific institutional and structural factors that increase the vulnerability of certain groups and that undermine their human capital accumulation. Such an understanding defines a clear and relevant research agenda for the future.

Chapter 6
Income and Health-Care Insecurity Among the Mexican-Origin Elderly

In the presentation we have taken a life-course perspective and investigated the ways in which parental occupational disadvantages affect children and how they affect health-care access and retirement plans for Mexican-origin adult men and women. Following the life-course logic, we now address the situation of older Hispanics. Given our focus on retirement and health benefits, we begin by examining the situation of individuals approaching retirement, as well as those of retirement age. As we show, the low incomes and lack of health and retirement plans that we documented among younger workers in earlier chapters have serious negative implications for the retirement security of older Hispanic men and women. Without the accumulated assets and the savings that a high income makes possible, older individuals with mixed work histories find themselves dependent on Social Security for income and Medicare alone for health care. Although Social Security and Medicare provide a badly needed safety net for older individuals with nothing else, they can leave an older individual or couple in danger of serious economic hardship or incomplete health care.

Retired individuals with low incomes and little wealth are in no position to help children buy homes, they are unable to contribute to higher education for grandchildren, and they face very limited consumption possibilities themselves. For many poor elderly individuals, regardless of their race or ethnicity, the retirement years are anything but golden. In this chapter, we examine the late-life consequences of the earlier-life occupational disadvantages that we have documented for Hispanic men and women 55 years of age and older. As we have illustrated in earlier chapters, in the United States employer-sponsored health insurance represents the largest source of health-care coverage for the working-age population. When one reaches the age of 65, though, one becomes eligible for Medicare, a program of universal basic health care for the elderly. Although the United States, unlike other developed nations, has never adopted a national health-care financing plan for everyone, the importance of health care among the elderly and their clear risk of destitution or inadequate care in the event of a medical crisis led to the passage of Medicare in 1965. In 2007, slightly more than 13.8% of insured Americans were covered by Medicare, and an additional 13.2% received Medicaid (DeNavas-Walt et al. 2008). As we will explain in detail later, Medicaid is a major source of supplemental

R.J. Angel, J.L. Angel, *Hispanic Families at Risk*, DOI 10.1007/978-1-4419-0474-4_6,

medical-care coverage and long-term care coverage for poor older Americans, and it is a very important program for older Hispanics.

Social Security and Medicare, then, have transformed the situation of the elderly, including African-American and Hispanic elderly. Today the lack of health-care coverage and very low incomes are concentrated among younger age groups, primarily working-age adults who do not qualify for public programs. Social Security, Medicare, and Medicaid have been crucial in preserving the legitimacy and viability of the employment-based health-care financing system of the United States. They addressed the most serious needs of two of the most potentially vulnerable segments of the population, the elderly and children. High rates of extreme poverty among either group would lay bare the inhumanity of an entirely privatized system and potentially undermine our political stability. Older individuals vote and organizations such as the American Association of Retired Persons (AARP) represent formidable political forces. Even a president as popular as Ronald Regan was unable to add a surcharge to the Medicare payments of affluent seniors over their well-organized and vociferous objections (Moon and Herd 2003; Oberlander 2001).

The issues and problems we identify among older Hispanics in this chapter are by definition different, then, than those we identified for children or working-age adults. After the age of 65 all US citizens and those legal residents who have been in the United States for at least 5 years who paid into Medicare for a minimum of 40 fiscal quarters, or 10 years, are eligible for Medicare (Centers for Medicare and Medicaid Services 2008). These individuals and their spouses qualify for Medicare Part A, which covers Hospital costs and they have the option of enrolling in Part B, which covers physician and other medical charges. With both Part A and Part B Medicare, older persons are guaranteed a fairly generous set of medical and hospital services at a time in life when health problems begin to accumulate (Eichner and Vladeck 2005). One might imagine, therefore, that after 65 years the negative association between minority status and health insurance coverage would disappear even for the Mexican-origin population, which as we saw at earlier ages is seriously underinsured and uninsured.

Clearly, Medicare is a major benefit for older Hispanics, as it is for all older Americans. Along with Social Security, Medicare has greatly decreased serious poverty and the lack of medical care for all groups. In addition, for the poorest older individuals Medicaid helps pay for Medicare premiums, long-term care, and other expenses that accompany serious physical and mental decline. Unfortunately, even with these public programs, low-income older individuals and couples face the possibility of financial ruin as the result of health-care costs that Medicare does not cover (Jacoby et al. 2001). The reality is that older individuals need supplemental insurance, usually referred to as Medigap, to cover the costs of services and care that Medicare does not pay. These include routine dental care and dental appliances, most extended long-term care, routine assistance with problems with activities of daily living (ADLs), alternative medicine, experimental procedures and treatments, acupuncture, most chiropractic services, care received outside of the United States cosmetic surgery, hearing aids, some preventive care such as immunizations, non-medical service such as private hospital rooms, and nonemergency transportation

(Medicare Rights Center 2008). Medical expenses not covered by Medicare can represent a serious financial burden to an older individual or couple on a limited income, and those who do not have supplemental Medigap plans face the risk of large medical debt or having to do without needed care.

Sixty-five, then, does not represent an age at which group-specific economic and health-care vulnerabilities disappear. There is no doubt that Social Security and Medicare greatly decrease the most serious inequalities and alleviate the most serious disadvantages among older Americans, but given lifelong differences in opportunities to accumulate wealth, it is not surprising that inequities in access to care, just as inequities in material welfare, persist into old age. We begin then by reviewing the sources of economic security among the elderly. As important as Social Security is in securing the economic well-being of the elderly, it is only one of what social security experts refer to as the three pillars of retirement security (Crystal 1982; Myles 1984). Social Security, which was never meant to be an older individual's sole source of income, is one of those pillars and perhaps the most important for poor Americans. The framers of Social Security intended for it to supplement the two other pillars, namely assets and private retirement plans (Quadagno and Street 2006). Unfortunately, as we saw in earlier chapters, individuals in low-wage occupations do not have the capacity to save, and even when they do have 401(k) plans, those plans remain badly underfunded. Intended or not, then, Social Security is the only source of income for many older individuals and, as we will see, this is often the case for Hispanics.

Those individuals who are in the strongest economic position in later life are those with a large stock of accumulated or inherited wealth. Wealth represents an individual and group asset that gives political and social power to groups and that gives individuals the ability to control important aspects of one's lives. For most Americans their home represents their major asset (Schulz and Binstock 2006). As is the case for 401(k) retirement plans, the recession of 2008 has seriously undermined the value of that asset, a tragedy that again affects those with the least amount of resources. In addition to owning more expensive houses, the wealthy have many other sources of economic security and power including cash, real estate, stocks, bonds, and other investments. In poor communities in which individuals have little human capital, few individuals inherit any significant amount and few are able to invest in wealth-generating ventures either on their own or in partnership with other community members. Despite the higher home ownership rate among the older population (71% for elderly singles and 93% for couple-headed households), the economic downturn has placed as many as 45% of all seniors at risk of financial hardship (Meschede et al. 2009). Although we all wish to live long lives, the downside is that we may outlive our resources.

The third pillar upon which economic security is based consists of private retirement plans. As we have shown in previous chapters, those group characteristics and labor market factors that result in low incomes are also associated with a lack of employment-based retirement coverage. In terms of the three pillars of income security in old age, then, Hispanics and other minorities are at a clear disadvantage in at least two, namely wealth and private retirement coverage. Even in terms of Social Security, though, they remain disadvantaged. Although Social Security is progressive in what it pays out to retirees in that individuals who had low incomes during their working lives receive a larger fraction of what they contributed as benefits, low-income workers receive smaller stipends than high-wage workers (Tanner 2005).

Medicare and Medicaid might well be included as a fourth pillar of economic security, although we do not usually think of these as income support programs. Given the high cost of medical care, which in the absence of Medicare and Medicaid would have to be paid for from some other source, these programs clearly have income support aspects. As an individual grows older he or she needs more medical care, and Medicare has clearly contributed to the economic well-being of the elderly by paying for much of that care. In this chapter, then, we draw on available national data, the literature on the economic and health situation of older Hispanics, an ongoing longitudinal study of the older Mexican-American population of the Southwest that is now in its 15th year, and the 2006 Health and Retirement Study (HRS), which includes an oversample of Hispanics, the majority of whom are of Mexican origin to characterize the situation of Hispanics in the later years of the life course. In order to understand the situation of Hispanics in the traditional retirement years, we begin our examination in the years just prior to retirement when an individual and couples assets and retirement possibilities are probably at their maximum.

Preretirement-Age Hispanics: Asset Poor

Since Social Security was introduced in 1935, poverty among the elderly has declined dramatically (Engelhardt and Gruber 2004). Today rates of poverty are higher for children in poor families than for those over 65 years (DeNavas-Walt et al. 2008). There can be little doubt that in the absence of Social Security, a large fraction of minority Americans would sink into poverty. The situation of older adults and older Hispanics, in particular, is best understood in terms of a life-course perspective in which an individual's economic and insurance situation in later life is related to the nature and course of his or her working life. A central debate concerning the old-age welfare state and income inequality among the elderly focuses on the question as to whether the inequalities that are so extreme among younger age groups persist into old age or whether Social Security and Medicare equalize differences among different groups. The answer to the question largely depends on the degree of equality in income and other assets that one considers significant. Social Security and Medicare have substantially reduced the worst poverty among the elderly and have provided them with basic medical care. Public programs have not eliminated, and clearly could not eliminate, the gap in wealth. In addition to persistent differences in wealth, as we show below, significant differences in income and medical-care coverage remain, in the case of health-care coverage largely as the result of Medigap coverage among the poor.

In order to better understand the situation of older Hispanics in retirement, then, we begin by examining their income and insurance situations in the years just before retirement and then move on to examine differences during the retirement years. To do so we employ the Health and Retirement Survey (HRS), a longitudinal study of the economic situation of individuals who were 51–61 years when the first wave of data were collected in 1992. The study includes oversamples of African-Americans and Hispanics, which makes it useful for our purposes (Juster and Suzman 1995). The panel was interviewed several more times after 1992 and new cohorts were added in 1998 and 2004. In our presentation, we use the first 1992 wave and the final 2006 wave. In this study, the researchers collected detailed information on health insurance as well as other employment, economic, and health information for single individuals and couples, at least one of whom was in the study age range. Unfortunately, the number of Cuban-Americans, Puerto Ricans, and other Hispanics is simply too small to support separate analyses or even the estimation of stable coefficients in pooled analyses. Rather than dropping them from the analysis or pooling them with Mexican-Americans as is commonly done, we treat them as a separate pooled category in the analysis for comparative purposes.

Wealth

Figure 6.1 presents data on the total value of the assets owned by non-Hispanic white, African-American, Mexican-origin, and other Hispanic households from the first wave of the HRS. We present the information separately for households headed by a male or a married couple and for female-headed households. Female headship represents a major dimension of economic disadvantage given the traditionally lower lifetime earnings of women and the fact that many have not been continuously employed. Female heads of household include those women who never married, those who are divorced, and widows. These women are likely to be in different economic situations, but unfortunately we do not have large-enough samples to examine their situations separately by race and ethnicity. Even the pooled data are informative, though, and it clearly reveals the serious wealth disadvantage associated with the combination of minority status and female headship. This figure reveals stark

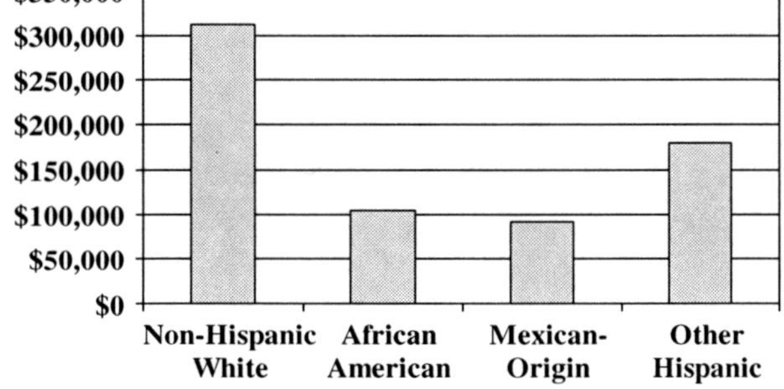

Fig. 6.1 Racial and ethnic group differences in male/couple-headed household wealth among preretirement-age individuals, 1992
Source: (Angel and Angel 2006)

differences in the total value of assets between minority and non-Hispanic households, as well as between those headed by a couple or a male and those headed by a female. In the years prior to retirement, non-Hispanic white male or couple-headed households had over $300,000 in total assets, whereas the average Mexican-origin couple had less than $100,000 in wealth. African-American couples were similarly asset poor. Other Hispanic couple-headed household were better off with approximately $200,000 in assets.

Female-headed households in all groups were seriously asset poor. Figure 6.2 shows that in most cases female-headed households had less than half the wealth of couple-headed households. Even though other Hispanic couple-headed households fare somewhat better than Mexican-origin or African-American couple-headed households, female-headed other Hispanic households have the least wealth of any group. It is clear, then, that minority status and gender represent two major dimensions of disadvantage, and that in combination they seriously undermine a household's economic security in later adulthood. Given such low levels of wealth one might imagine that minority Americans would choose to continue working or simply find that they have no choice but to do so. Based on estimates from the 2002 to 2005 Current Population Survery (CPS), 11% of older Hispanics continued working after the age of 65, compared with 13.6% of non-Hispanic whites (Finkle et al. 2007). These slightly lower rates may reflect the fact that Hispanics are more likely to have worked in physically demanding jobs in construction and agriculture that are difficult for older workers to perform. A professor might well continue working and receive a good salary until 70 even if he or she becomes somewhat frail, but a farm worker cannot continue working if his or her health declines. Given longer life spans and the economic crisis, though, employment rates among the elderly, including Hispanics, may well increase in the years to come. Analyses of employment patterns among the elderly suggest that retirement for older Hispanics is not the voluntary termination of a career but rather the involuntary end of a long period of unstable employment. Such a career trajectory is one that results in inadequate asset accumulation and a high risk of late-life poverty (Flippen and Tienda 2000).

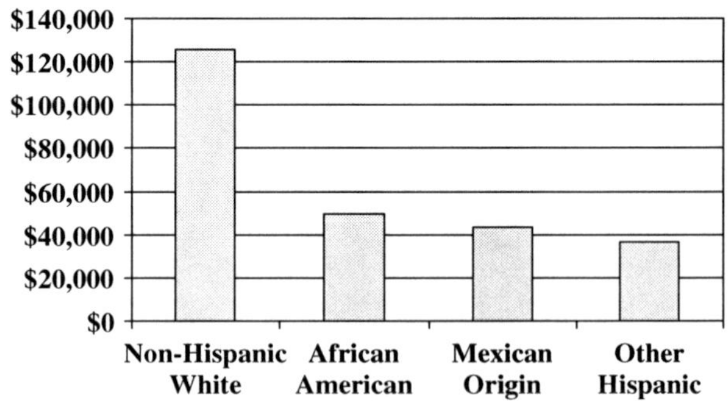

Fig. 6.2 Racial and ethnic group differences in female-headed household wealth among preretirement-age individuals, 1992 *Source*: (Angel and Angel 1996).

These differences in total household assets are striking and call for a bit more elaboration. Figure 6.3 provides a comparison of the total wealth of native-born

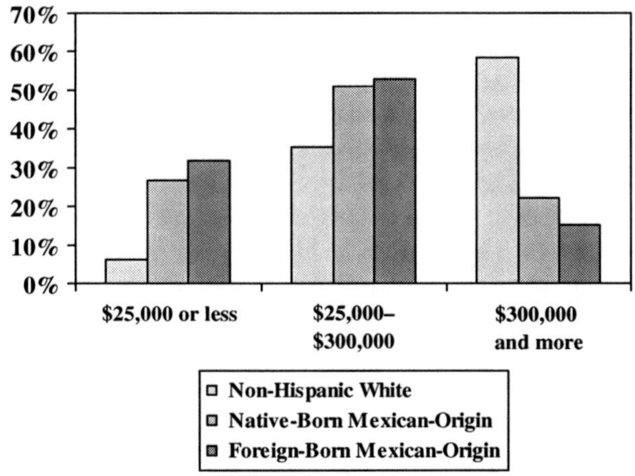

Fig. 6.3 Wealth of elderly couple-headed households by race and Mexican Origin, 2006
Source: Health and Retirement Study (2006).

and foreign-born Mexican-origin couple-headed households from the 2006 wave of the HRS. In this figure, all heads of household are over 65. The difference in wealth between non-Hispanic white householders of retirement age and Mexican-origin householders is again striking, but the figure also reveals a significant effect of nativity. Foreign-born households are overrepresented in the lowest wealth category and underrepresented in the highest, although both groups have far less wealth than non-Hispanic white households. Figure 6.4 presents these same wealth data for female-headed household to illustrate the serious disadvantage associated with the combination of Mexican-origin and female. Again, non-Hispanic white female-headed households are substantially richer than Mexican-origin female-headed households, and the figure shows the serious wealth poverty among the foreign-born, nearly 60% of whom have less than $25,000 in assets.

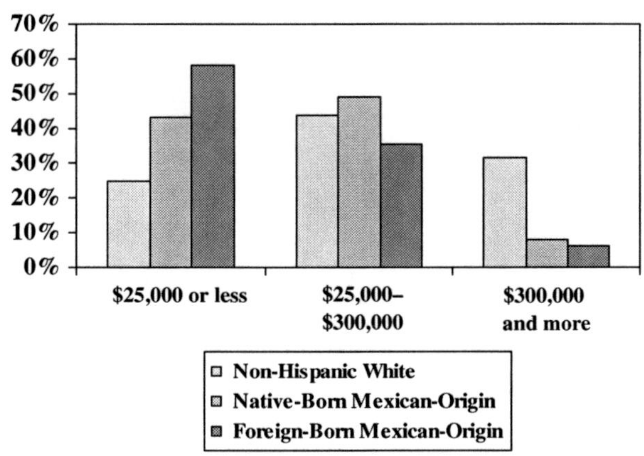

Fig. 6.4 Wealth of elderly female-headed households by race and Mexican Origin, 2006
Source: Health and Retirement Study (2006).

Income

These differences in wealth are highly significant since assets represent a major source of income for the most economically secure elderly individuals and couples. Returns on investments that have had years to grow, the sale of a business that one built into a profitable enterprise, or inheritances from wealthy parents differentiate the truly secure from those who just get by. Assets provide income in the form of interest payments or as capital gains when they are sold. For the majority of Americans, their home is their largest asset. Ideally, one should have paid off the mortgage by the time one retires so that the equity remains free and clear. If one needs cash for medial expenses, long-term care, or other purposes one can borrow against that equity or obtain a reverse mortgage, a product that allows one to sell one's home to a bank or other lender who pays the owner a set monthly amount based on the home's market value. In the absence of other assets, many individuals have no choice but to sell their home. Of course this means that one's estate is diminished and many people resist not leaving anything to their heirs, but again many simply have no choice and must liquidate what little they have.

As the previous section showed, racial and ethnic differences in wealth are huge by the time one approaches retirement years. These differences translate directly into racial and ethnic differences in income. Figure 6.5 presents data on sources of income for non-Hispanic white, African-American, and Hispanic individuals from the Social Security Administration for 2004. The bars indicate the proportion of each group that receives income from assets, pensions, or Social Security. The data show that while nearly half of non-Hispanic whites have asset income, only 23% of Hispanics report income from this source. In addition, while 31% of non-Hispanic whites report pension income, only half of that number of Hispanics reports pension income. For both assets and pensions, African-Americans are closer to Hispanics

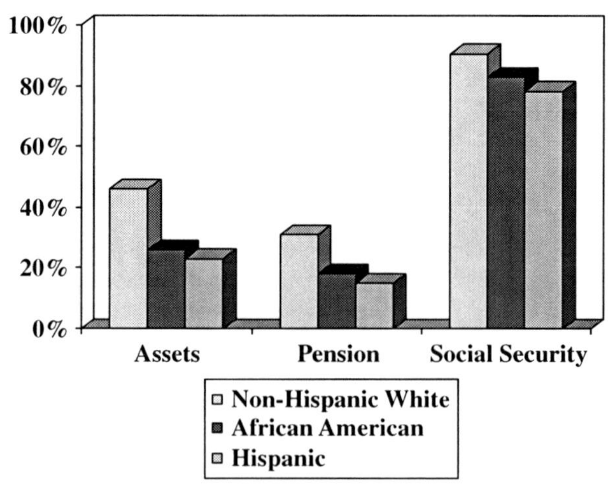

Fig. 6.5 Sources of retirement security in population aged 65 years and older, 2002
Source: Social Security Administration (2004b).

than non-Hispanic whites, revealing a clear minority dimension to these income sources. The figure clearly shows the universal importance of Social Security but still reveals a serious ethnic differential. While 91% of non-Hispanic whites receive Social Security, only 78% of Hispanics receive Social Security.

After wealth, private retirement plans represent a major source of income for retired individuals and couples. Without a private pension one must live on Social Security alone, which as we have shown provides a very modest income. As we discussed in Chapter 1, the major structural problem that affects the retirement income security of Hispanics results from the lack of retirement savings. Employment in low-wage jobs precludes adequate saving and few service-sector jobs offer retirement plans. In the United States, employers are not required to offer retirement plans. If an employer chooses to offer such a plan, usually through an insurance company, that plan must conform to federal laws concerning funding, vesting, and administration (Schulz and Binstock 2006). In the absence of a mandate to cover workers, the cost of offering such a plan discourages marginal employers from offering one. This is particularly true for the small service-sector employers who employ Mexican-origin workers. As a consequence, older Hispanics are far less likely than other groups to have private pension plans. According to the National Council of La Raza, 75% of Hispanics have no retirement coverage compared to 50% of the population at large (National Council of La Raza 2004).

In addition to lower participation rates, Hispanics who participate in employer-sponsored 401(k) plans contribute less than other groups. The average value of 401(k) plans among Hispanic households with incomes from $50,000 to 75,000 with such plans is only one-half of the average for all households ($23,000 versus $58,000). Mexican-origin workers, especially the foreign-born, are less likely than non-Hispanic workers to have access to retirement planning services, financing counseling, and advice concerning investing and savings (National Council of La Raza 2005a). In addition to low wages and inadequate information concerning planning and saving, a large fraction Mexican-origin families fail to save adequately for retirement. Proposals for private investment accounts or even a partial privatization of Social Security are unlikely to improve the situation of families with few resources and little knowledge of investing (National Council of La Raza 2005b). Low levels of savings and the lack of retirement plans, then, mean that elderly Mexican-origin individuals rely disproportionately on social security and other assistance programs. Approximately 13% of Hispanics aged 65 and over receive Supplemental Security Income (SSI), compared with only 3% of elderly non-Hispanic whites and 10% of African-Americans of the same age (Social Security Administration 2005).

Figure 6.6 presents information from the 2006 HRS concerning retirement income for native and foreign-born Mexican-origin family households in which the head is 65 or older. It shows that while 73% of non-Hispanic white households have a retirement plan of some sort, only 39% of native-born and 15% of foreign-born households have any retirement plan. The figure also compares Mexican-origin with non-Hispanic white households in terms of income from defined benefit plans or defined contribution plans (IRA/Keogh). The numbers add up to more than the "any

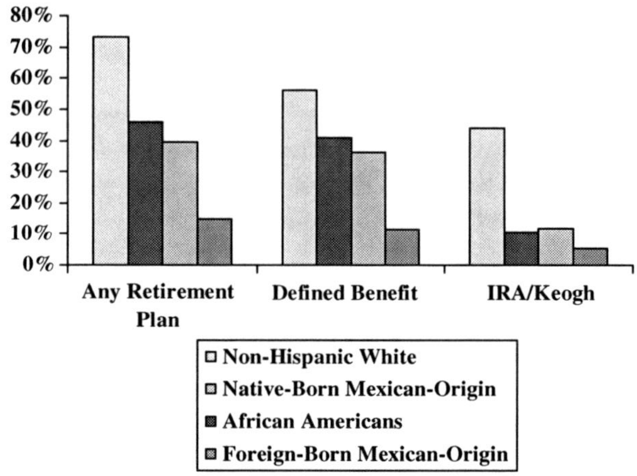

Fig. 6.6 Retirement plan of elderly household by race and Mexican Origin, 2006
Source: Health and Retirement Study (2006).

retirement plan column" since individuals can have both types of plan, usually from different employers. Again the figure reveals serious deficits for Mexican-origin households compared with non-Hispanic households, and especially for foreign-born households, only 11% of which have a defined-benefit plan and only 5% of which have a defined-contribution plan. It appears, then, only a minority of Mexican-origin households of retirement age is receiving income from this important income security pillar.

Social Security

Social Security retirement income (Old-Age and Survivors Insurance) is, of course, the major public income program for older Americans. It was designed to protect older Americans from severe poverty and it is vital to the large population of Mexican-origin elders who lack accumulated wealth or private retirement plans (Angel and Angel 1997). Given the universal nature of the program, nearly all retired Americans qualify and most participate (Achenbaum 1986).

However, certain Hispanics do not qualify for Social Security Retirement Income. Approximately 76% of Hispanics over the age of 62, the age at which one can retire with reduced benefits, receive social security retirement compared with 91% of non-Hispanic whites and 85% of non-Hispanic blacks (Fry et al. 2005). These statistics reflect the fact that a significant fraction of older Mexican-Americans, and especially among the foreign-born, do not receive benefits (Fry et al. 2005). There are several possible reasons for not receiving Social Security. Many Mexican-origin workers spent their lives engaged in non-covered employment, or they were employed only intermittently or seasonally. Many had multiple Social Security numbers and often their employers failed to make required contributions. When the Social Security program was introduced in 1935, agricultural and domestic workers, occupations that are disproportionately Hispanic and

African-American, were not included (Poole, 2006; Quadagno, 1994; Social Security Administration 2009). One major injustice in the system is that undocumented workers often pay taxes during their work lives but do not collect benefits that they are entitled to because they fear government reprisal (Smith and Edmonston 1997). Anti-immigrant sentiments which have grown in recent years have had a chilling effect that discourages entitled immigrants to ask for services or apply for benefits (de la Garza 2005).

Social Security is the major source of income for perhaps over half of older Mexican-origin retirees. Forty-four percent of Hispanics in the United States rely on Social Security for at least 90% of their income compared with 29% of non-Hispanic whites (Hendley and Bilimoria 1999). Without Social Security, over half of elderly Hispanics would live in poverty (Torres-Gil et al. 2005). Yet even with Social Security, older Hispanics face a fairly austere retirement. In 2005 the average Social Security benefit for all beneficiaries was $9,900, but for Hispanics it was only $8,056 (Martin 2007). Individuals who rely solely on Social Security have little discretionary income and face difficulties paying for other expenses, including those for medical care that are not covered by Medicare (Grossman et al. 2008).

As a result of an exclusive dependence on a minimal Social Security income, many Mexican-origin elders remain in poverty, or precariously close to it, and their retirement years are plagued by economic uncertainty (Torres-Gil et al. 2005). A 1997 survey by the Pew Charitable Trusts shows that approximately one-third of Hispanics who are not currently poor fear that they will descend into poverty in old age. Only one-fifth of non-Hispanic whites and African-Americans share that fear (Princeton Survey Research Associates 1998). A 2005 survey of Hispanic retirees show that 40% of foreign-born Hispanics believed the social security system has severe problems (i.e., "in crisis or faced major problems") compared with close to 60% of native-born Hispanics (Fry et al. 2005).

Health Insurance

The data clearly show that Hispanics have less wealth and lower incomes than non-Hispanic whites as they approach and enter the retirement years. There can be little doubt that they are seriously disadvantaged in terms of all three of the major income security pillars. This lack of wealth and income has serious consequences for individuals, families, and the Hispanic community as a whole. The lack of collective assets means that there is less equity and savings available for individuals and businesses to draw upon for daily needs or to build a better future. As bad as the situation we have documented might be, it is even more serious when one considers health insurance coverage. As we mentioned earlier, given the importance of health care to older individuals it makes sense to think of health insurance or health-care coverage as a fourth pillar of economic security. Given the high prevalence of serious chronic health conditions among those over 65, health-care coverage has major income support aspects.

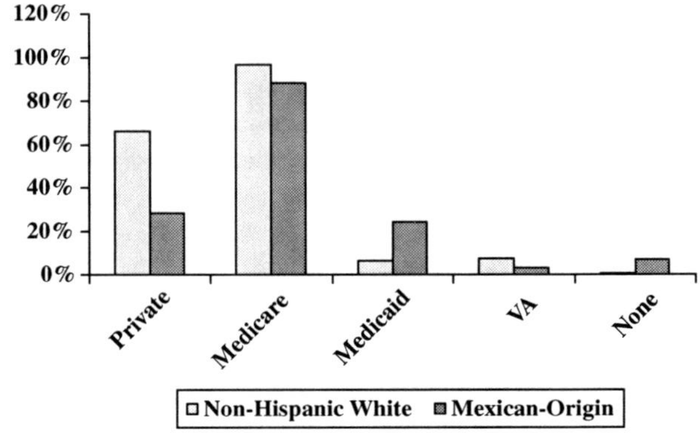

Fig. 6.7 Health insurance coverage for older adults by race and Hispanic ethnicity, 2006
Source: Current Population Survey (2004, 2006).

Figure 6.7 compares sources of health insurance coverage among non-Hispanic white and Mexican-origin individuals over 65 in 2006. In this figure, the private category includes supplemental Medigap plans either provided by a previous employer or purchased on the open market from such organizations as the American Association for Retired Persons (AARP) or insurance companies. The figure shows the high rates of Medicare coverage that result from the fact that the program is a universal entitlement. Nonetheless, it also shows that 12% of Mexican-origin elders do not participate or at least report that they do not participate. As in the case of wealth and income, Mexican-origin elderly fall far below non-Hispanic whites in terms of private Medigap coverage. Only 29% of Mexican-origin elders have such a policy, compared to 66% of non-Hispanic whites. This lack of Medigap coverage, combined with the low assets and wealth we have documented, means that a larger proportion of Mexican-origin elders receive Medicaid. For the destitute elderly, Medicaid covers Medicare premiums and other costs and also pays for long-term care. In order to qualify for Medicaid long-term care, one must "spend down" to the qualification level, which means that one has basically nothing left.

The lack of supplemental health insurance in old-age range places many of these individuals at serious risk of ill health and its longer term consequences (Schur et al. 1995). This is the point in the life course during which the consequences of chronic diseases, such as diabetes and hypertension which are very common in the Mexican-origin population, take their greatest toll (Markides et al. 1997). Among the Mexican-origin elderly, over 40% rely solely on Medicare. Although Medicare is clearly superior to no insurance, it requires a monthly premium, co-payments, deductibles for hospitalization, and more. In the absence of Medigap coverage, low-income older individuals may simply have to do without the medical care or the drugs they need.

As we have seen, then, the lack of health insurance is part of a package that includes low income and impaired asset accumulation. By the time an individual or a couple reach the ages of 51–61 years, they have accumulated most of the wealth that they will ever have. Homes are close to being paid off and one's income is as high as it will ever be. Differences in wealth between groups during the preretirement years mean large differences in economic well-being and health during retirement. These differences have particularly profound implications for options in long-term care. Low income and a lack of retirement health benefits place minority Americans at serious risk of dependency on family or of incomplete and inadequate health care in old age (Angel and Anbgel, 1996).

Overall, the data present a bleak picture in terms of economic well-being among preretirement-age black, Hispanics, and single women. It is unlikely that the economic situations of individuals over age 50 will improve dramatically and when they reach their 70s and 80s many blacks, Hispanics, and single women will have very few assets to draw upon if they need long-term care. Due to the double jeopardy of gender and minority group status, the situation of single black men and Hispanic minority women is particularly precarious.

The Lack of Medigap Coverage

To assess health-care coverage among older Mexican-origin individuals, we employ data from a longitudinal study carried out in the Southwestern United States (Angel et al. 2002a). The study, entitled the Hispanic Established Population for Epidemiologic Studies of the Elderly (Hispanic-EPESE), has followed a cohort of 3,050 Mexican-origin individuals who were 65 years or older and who lived in Arizona, California, Colorado, New Mexico, and Texas at the time of the first interview in 1993 and 1994. Detailed information on household demographics, economics, health status, and health-care use was collected. The sample was recontacted and much of the same information collected again in 1995–1996, 1998–1999, and 2000–2001. At each wave, information on individuals who were too incapacitated to respond for themselves was collected from a knowledgeable proxy. Nearly half of the sample was foreign-born and more than half had household incomes below the poverty level.

Figure 6.8 presents information on health insurance coverage in this relatively poor sample of older Mexican-Americans. It shows that the Mexican-origin elderly are particularly dependent on Medicaid and that only 19% have private Medigap plans; 41% depend on Medicare alone. The lack of supplemental coverage places these individuals at serious risk of not receiving the care they need (Angel and Angel 1997). Medicare physician coverage requires the payment of a monthly premium, and a substantial fair-share cost is associated with hospital stays. In addition, Medicare does not cover the cost of prescription drugs, eyeglasses, hearing aids, or other specialized medical devices and appliances. The costs of a medical encounter for an older person without supplemental coverage can be quite high. As at other ages, the lack of a supplemental Medigap plan is part of a package that includes a lifetime of employment in jobs that do not provide retirement health plans and a retirement income that can make the purchase of private coverage prohibitively expensive.

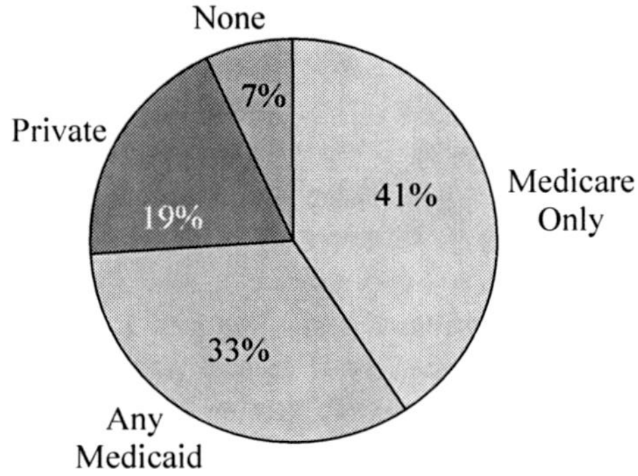

Fig. 6.8 Health insurance coverage for older Mexican-Americans in the Southwestern United States, 1994
Source: Hispanic EPESE (1993–1994).

Medicaid represents the health-care safety net for the poor elderly. For those with incomes below or slightly above poverty, Medicaid covers the costs of premiums and other costs associated with Medicare. Such individuals have come to be referred to as "dual eligible" because they qualify for both Medicare and Medicaid. Dual eligibility, therefore, is itself an indicator of vulnerability. Unfortunately, for those individuals with incomes above 200% of poverty, Medicaid is not available and if they do not have a private Medigap plan, these older individuals must rely on their own resources to pay for what Medicare will not. For that reason, the accumulated assets are particularly important.

What is particularly striking about Fig. 6.8 is that 7% of these elderly Mexican-origin respondents report no health insurance of any kind, a figure higher than that for the nation as a whole (cf. Fig. 6.7). These data then reflect the unique disadvantage of those older individuals living along the U.S. Mexico border. To make some sense of these findings, we present type of health insurance by nativity and life course stage at migration in Table 6.1. Among late-life migrants almost 30% report no insurance and only 5.2% report that they have any private Medigap insurance; 35% are dual eligible. The data show, then, that nativity interacts with region

Table 6.1 Type of health insurance coverage by nativity and age at migration for elderly Mexican-Americans: 1993–1994 (weighted percent; unweighted *N*'s in parentheses)

Age at migration	No insurance	Medicare only	Any Medicaid	Private[1]
Late-life	29.8	30.6	34.5	5.2
Middle age	6.1	46.6	31.6	15.8
Childhood	6.7	40.3	33.0	20.1
Native Born	3.2	38.7	26.5	31.6
Sample size	(137)	(1,205)	(958)	(634)

[1] Includes military health care, i.e., CHAMPUS (Comprehensive Health and Medical Plan for Uniformed Services), CHAMPVA (Civilian Health and Medical Program of the Department of Veteran's Affairs).
Source: H-EPESE.

and other factors to place Mexican-origin individuals in poorly paid service sector jobs in which they do not receive benefits. The disadvantage this group faces, therefore, arises from multiple sources and for a large fraction is lifelong. This hardened disadvantage presents policymakers with a serious challenge in providing adequate health-care coverage to the Mexican-origin population.

There are many possible reasons for these lower rates of nonparticipation in Medicare among older Mexican-origin individuals and for the lack of private Medigap insurance among Hispanics generally. For those of Mexican origin, citizenship status may represent a barrier. Many older Mexican-Americans have never have become legal residents of the United States. For those who do not speak English, which is quite common among older cohorts, access problems may keep them from seeking medical care or participating in Social Security. Among younger age groups, lower rates of participation in Medicaid are largely accounted for by the restrictive participation criteria imposed by states such as Texas and Florida. Among the elderly, for whom Medicare is a universal entitlement, state-imposed eligibility barriers are less serious and other access factors become more salient.

What the data show, then, is that the vast majority of older Hispanics participate in the Medicare program (Angel and Angel 2006). However, as Fig. 6.7 and Fig. 6.8 show, a small but significant percent report that they have no health insurance coverage of any kind. Older Mexican-origin individuals are less likely than non-Hispanic whites to have supplemental Medigap coverage and rely solely on Medicare with Medicaid as a backup (Angel and Angel 2006). Supplemental insurance is necessary since Medicare involves premiums, co-payments, and cost sharing for hospital stays, and it does not cover the cost of all services. Some estimates indicate that low-income Medicare beneficiaries spend an average of 35% of their income on out-of-pocket health expenses (Texas Department on Aging 2002). Out-of-pocket payments associated with Medicare pose a particular hardship for older Mexican-origin individuals with limited economic resources, especially those in Texas border counties. Since Medicare reimbursements to doctors are low, many physicians limit the number of Medicare patients they take and elderly Mexican-origin beneficiaries may have difficulty finding a doctor or they may receive a lower level of health care than others (Angel et al. 2002b).

Medicare Advantage, a new program that allows groups of physicians to offer bundled services to clients, may benefit poor Mexican-origin elders, even if the program itself is criticized for its high cost. The value of Medicare Advantage to Mexican-origin elder beneficiaries stems from the fact that it provides access to private plans in states with large rural elderly Mexican-origin populations, including Texas and California. Because these programs are more affordable for low-income elders and include benefits not found in traditional fee-for-serve Medicare, many low-income elderly Mexican-Americans benefit from them (Atherly and Thorpe 2005). Forty percent of African-American and 53% of Hispanic beneficiaries without Medicaid or employer coverage rely on Medicare Advantage, compared with 33% of non-Hispanic white beneficiaries.

Long-Term Care

The debate over who should bear the financial and practical responsibility for frail older adults continues more than 70 years after the Social Security Act was passed. Throughout most of human history, older individuals have been cared for by their families, often in extended multigeneration households. This is particularly the case for elderly Hispanics who are the least likely to use nursing homes, as shown in Fig. 6.9. Since Social Security was introduced, children no longer expect to assume the full financial responsibility for their aging parents. In effect, basic financial security in old age has been socialized. Long-term care services are a major exception. Unlike medical and short-term hospital care, nursing home and other ongoing care are not available to everyone at public expense. Publicly funded long-term care remains means-tested and available only to older individuals with very low incomes who have spent all of their savings and liquidated their assets. For those who do become destitute, Medicaid serves as the long-term care safety net of last resort. While the debate over who should receive Social Security is settled, the debate over who should receive Medicaid-financed long-term care and how extensive the services offered should be remains an issue of intense debate (Schulz and Binstock 2006).

Given the low levels of lifetime asset accumulation we have documented, and their relatively low wages, means-tested programs such as Medicaid are critical for the elderly Hispanic population. In order to illustrate the nature of the old-age welfare state and its role in the lives of frail and disabled older Hispanics in what follows we describe the major long-term care programs for the elderly in the United States and focus on Texas, a state with a large Mexican-origin population and a limited welfare state. Unless one is an expert, one probably is not familiar with the details of long-term care financing so we briefly explain the role of Medicaid in paying for long-term care for impoverished older individuals who can no longer care for themselves. It is important to understand how the eligibility criteria and coverage levels differentially affect the Mexican-origin population. As we will show, some aspects of the design of these programs potentially result in reduced benefits for the elderly Mexican-origin population.

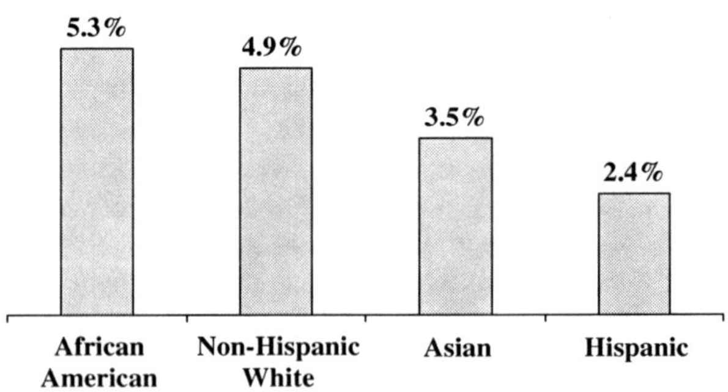

Fig. 6.9 Institutionalized population aged 65 years and over by race/Hispanic ethnicity, 2000
Source: (Angel and Hogan, 2004).

Medicaid and Long-Term Care

Medicaid is the funder of last resort for both acute and long-term care for poor Americans. It is particularly important in states such as California and Texas which have large Hispanic populations mostly of Mexican-origin, of whom large fractions are immigrants. Medicaid receipt among the foreign-born is common. Almost two-thirds of Mexican-origin individuals 65 years and over in Texas who immigrated after age 50 relied on Medicaid coverage in 1993 and 1994 (Angel 2003). Similar patterns emerge in California where approximately 40% of older Mexican-origin adults who immigrated in mature adulthood receive Medicaid (Angel 2003). For adults with very low incomes, Medicaid pays the premium for Part B, physician and medical services, and covers other costs. Most importantly, though, Medicaid pays for long-term care in nursing homes and other facilities for individuals who either have almost no income or assets, or who have "spent down," a term used to refer to a situation in which an older person is essentially broke. The program covers citizens and legal residents who have been in the United States for 5 years or more.

Given their larger families and preference for staying in the community, a relatively small proportion of even very frail older Mexican-origin individuals use nursing homes (Angel et al. 2004). Changes in the Mexican-origin family, though, may signal the end of its ability to support an infirm older individual at home (Angel and Hogan 2004; Angel and Angel 2006). Perhaps the most important change affecting the family's ability to care for older parents is the decline in the availability of daughters or daughters-in-law to provide care. As we noted in the last chapter, women, including Hispanic women, find it necessary to enter the labor force, often because there is no male in the house. Traditionally, women were the primary caregivers for older parents and in-laws, but by 2004, 69.5% of Mexican-origin women aged 25–54 years were employed full time (U.S. Department of Labor 2005). With their new responsibilities outside of the home they have less time to devote to caregiving, especially for older relatives who require round-the-clock care. In the future, declining fertility rates will further decrease the number of family members available to care for the elderly.

This decline in the family's caregiving capacity comes at a time when the proportion of the Mexican-origin population, as is the case with all groups, is growing relative to the number of younger individuals. In Texas over the next 40 years, the relative size of the general population aged 65 and over will double relative to the population of 16- to 64-year-olds (Texas State Data Center 2006). In 2000 individuals aged 60 and older made up 13% of the population of Texas. By 2040 they will make up almost one quarter of the state's total population (Texas Department of Aging 2003).

Despite the fact that Texas' fertility remains higher than other states, Texas has the second largest number of Hispanics aged 60 and over in the nation, making up almost 20% of the general older population (Texas Department of Aging 2003). Demographers project that the percentage of Hispanics aged 65 and older will increase three-fold from 6.4% in 2006 to 17.5% in 2050 (Federal Interagency Forum on Aging-Related Statistics 2008). The state also anticipates as the result of the declining birth rate, that a larger fraction, perhaps as much as 15%, of Hispanic baby boomers will remain childless, translating into a growing older population without children to depend on for support (Murdock et al. 2002). For the moment, though, Mexican-origin families remain larger than those of other racial and ethnic groups and they continue to provide the care that older members need.

In the absence of a community support system, however, frail older Mexican-origin individuals who are unable to manage in their own homes, and those who have depleted whatever resources they possess, have no recourse but Medicaid-funded long-term care. One bit of potentially good news is that such care can be provided in the community, and for those who would like to stay close to their familiar surroundings but who could not do so without formal assistance, the option may be ideal. As a matter of fact, given the option most elderly individuals prefer to remain in their own homes and communities for as long as possible. Cost studies of community options provide evidence that many home- and community-based programs can provide services at a cost comparable to that provided in nursing homes (Kitchener et al. 2006; Ladd et al. 1995). Community-based options are still not the norm though and Texas spends less on community-based care than on nursing homes. The state now spends only one dollar in alternative care programs for every $2.33 spent on nursing home care (Stevenson et al. 2006). The option for community care is particularly important for older Mexican-origin elders who have community supports but find that those are inadequate to provide all of the care they need. The aging of the population at a time when informal family-based support structures are coming under greater strain means that alternative means of providing services in cost-effective ways must be explored.

As important as Medicaid is for poor Hispanic elderly, the program faces ongoing political challenges related to financing because of the fact that it is a joint federal/state program to which the state must contribute. Today Medicaid consumes a large fraction of state budgets, and as the population ages and a greater number of older individuals exhaust their resources, state budgets will come under increasing strain. The growing cost makes Medicaid a major point of contention in state legislatures (Schulz and Binstock 2006). Generous programs may benefit the elderly, but they come at the cost of other projects and programs that states wish to pursue, including primary, secondary, and higher education. Since Mexican-origin elders have far fewer resources to use to pay for long-term case, the role of Medicaid and other public programs becomes particularly salient.

In addition to improving an older person's quality of life, community alternatives might be designed to be less expensive than high-level nursing home care. In order to explore these community options, Texas has applied for and received several home- and community-based Medicaid waivers that offer alternatives to nursing homes. Waivers are part of federal legislation that allow states to experiment with new ways of providing social services, under the condition that the experimental programs cost no more than the existing program. Community-based programs initiated under the waiver authority serve as laboratories for testing cost-neutral ways of packaging services and reimbursing providers. These Medicaid-community-based programs encompass a wide array of services that help meet the needs of older Texans with disabilities, including but not limited to adult foster care, home-delivered meals, respite care, primary home care, and day activity and health services.

In general, the evidence suggests that these programs could be operated more economically than institutionally based options, especially on a statewide basis (Lewin Group 2004; Rudolph and Lubitz 1999). Currently, community services are unavailable in many areas of the state and many programs have long waiting lists. According to the Texas House Research Organization, at least 47,000 Texans are on the state's waiting lists for Medicaid long-term care community-based waiver programs, where some nursing home residents have remained for more than 10 years (Texas House of Representatives 2005).

A closer examination of one waiver program would help illustrate their potential utility for the older Mexican-origin population in Texas. The Bienvivir ("Live Well" in Spanish) Centers which are part of an initiative entitled "Program for All Inclusive Care for the Elderly" are particularly well-suited for older Mexican-origin individuals for several reasons. First, the program is located in El Paso in a county that is over 80% Hispanic. Second, the program's age-eligibility criterion, 55 and older, better reflects the age structure of the Mexican-origin population which includes a younger elderly population than the nation as a whole. Third, the program model helps frail seniors maintain or improve function in order to allow them to live independently in the community with some family assistance. This special feature includes comprehensive medical and social services using an interdisciplinary team approach in an adult day health center that is supplemented by in-home and referral services with the client's preferences in mind.

For elderly Mexican-Americans such community-based support programs mean that family members who live close by can interact with them on a regular basis without being overly burdened. Texas views the El Paso experiment as an ideal model which may save the state long-term care dollars for the growing older Mexican-origin population. The average monthly cost of participants in 2006 was $2,028 in El Paso compared with nursing home totals of $2,817 in Houston and $2,817 in Dallas/Ft. Worth (U.S. Office of Personnel Management 2008). The El Paso program, then, demonstrates the possibility of taking advantage of group-specific characteristics, in this case larger families, to design new ways of providing needed support to older individuals who might otherwise be forced into undesirable situations.

In addition to Medicaid-funded long-term care services, other programs provide services that older individuals need in order to remain in the community. These home- and community-based services include benefits counseling, care coordination, caregiver support, information and referral, nutritional meals, and legal assistance (Alamo Area Council of Governments 2007). In San Antonio, which is located in Bexar County, the Bexar Area Agency on Aging provides a good example of novel ways of providing assistance to older Mexican-origin elders. The City of San Antonio takes up 80% of Bexar County and ranks seventh in population among cities in the United States (U.S. Census Bureau 2006a). The Bexar Area Agency on Agency's clientele is 43% Hispanic origin, the largest percent of which represents people aged 60 and older of Mexican ancestry (Alamo Area Council of Governments 2007).

Compared to other urban areas in the state, a larger percentage of the county's residents, especially those of Mexican-origin, are poor, unemployed, and have low levels of education (Alamo Area Council of Governments 2007). For young working families who must care for their aging parents, the combination of factors can result in significant hardship and financial sacrifice (Leland, 2009).

The projected growth in the 60 and older and minority population in Bexar County may seriously strain resources and require a reduction of services. Although many older people need modifications to their dwellings to accommodate disabilities, because of the high cost it is increasingly difficult for Area Agencies on Aging to build ramps and perform other minor home modifications. Homemaker services are another key service in the community that is increasingly difficult to provide. For example, at the Bexar Area Agency on Aging, waiting lists for homemaker and personal care services have at times grown to as many as 500 applicants (Alamo Area Council of Governments 2007).

Information and Outreach for Older Adults

Lower rates of supplemental Medigap coverage among Mexican-origin seniors mean that many lack access to the full range of services they need. For this reason, it is important that all low-income seniors receive information about the state assistance programs for which they may qualify. Currently, several programs help pay Medicare premiums, deductibles, and coinsurance for eligible low-income Medicare beneficiaries. The most generous is the Qualified Medicare Beneficiaries (QMB) program, which pays Medicare Part A and B premiums, deductibles, and coinsurance. As is the case for all programs with state contributions, states vary in qualification criteria and amount paid. To qualify for this program in Texas, an individual must have a very modest income, less than $736 per month. As with programs for children, outreach efforts can increase participation among those who are eligible.

Recent efforts by the Texas Department on Aging and Disability Services (DADS) to increase access to Medicaid services for "dual eligible" Hispanic retirees, a term that refers to those older individuals who receive Medicare but who are also eligible for Medicaid because of low income, along the US-Mexico border suggest that state and local partnerships that include community- and faith-based organizations and other nongovernmental agencies, and that employ bilingual outreach specialists, can increase enrollment (Stockton et al. 2001). As has been demonstrated with programs for children, administrative streamlining also helps. Making the application process easier, including a Spanish language version of a single application that combines eligibility requirements for both federal and state programs, would likely increase the number of elderly Mexican-Americans who apply (Carliner 2002).

Future Possibilities and Limitations

In the coming years, the United States will be faced with the reality of having to address the needs of a rapidly growing racially and ethnically diverse elderly population. As we mentioned in Chapter 2, the racial and ethnic diversity of states such as California and Texas intersects with the system of social stratification that determines where in the economic and social hierarchy older individuals from each group find themselves. In the United States an individual or couple's income and financial security in retirement depend on the principal wage earner's ability to save during his or her working life, as well as his or her access to an employer-sponsored retirement plan. As we have shown in this chapter, given the fact that ethnicity places Hispanics, and especially Mexican-origin workers, at a serious disadvantage in the labor market, a disproportionate number of these individuals and couples find themselves in dire economic straights in later life. During their working lives many Hispanics accumulate little wealth, have no or little private retirement coverage, and in retirement rely exclusively on Social Security and Medicare. These programs have clearly improved the lives of older Americans, including those of minority Americans. The vast majority of individuals are assured at least a limited retirement wage and Medicare assures access to basic medical care. Older Mexican-origin individuals, at least those who have become citizens or those who qualify for publicly sponsored social services, are better off in the United States than in Mexico. The challenge for the future will be to improve benefit coverage among younger workers so that their financial situation in old age is more secure. Additionally, the challenge will be to make sure that the inevitable cuts in Medicaid that the fiscal crisis makes necessary do not unfairly penalize those with the fewest resources.

Chapter 7
Segmented Labor Markets, Segmented Lives: Hispanic Workers and the Employment-Based Welfare State

The historic recession of 2008 clearly revealed the weakness of the employment-based health care and retirement financing systems upon which Americans have come to rely. The recession brought home to the middle class what has always been the reality for minority and low-wage Americans. In one year retirement savings plans lost almost half of their value and millions of Americans were thrown out of work. At the time this manuscript goes to press, the recession is a bit over a year old and the extent of the eventual damage will not be clear for some time. The recession was, of course, global and seriously affected the economies of all nations. All over the world workers lost their jobs and saw their personal savings erode, yet the differences in the impact of unemployment were stark. In the United States when workers lose their jobs they not only lose income, they lose their health-care coverage as well. Those who belong to an employer-sponsored group plan are by law allowed to continue their participation at their own expense for up to 18 months or more, but they must cover the full cost, which in 2008 was over $12,000 a year for a family policy (Kaiser Family Foundation 2008). In other developed nations, the loss of a job does not mean the loss of health-care coverage because of near universality of national health insurance.

No nation or government, no matter how generous in principle it might be, can guard everyone from all of the risks of life. Risk is inevitable and recessions, natural disasters, and personal setbacks occur at regular intervals. The fundamental problem that societies face has to do with how that risk is pooled. Since we have been dealing with health insurance we might continue with the insurance metaphor in discussing the moral dimensions of the welfare state. The core concept of insurance is the "risk pool," which refers to the number of individuals who participate and share the particular risk against which they are insured. During the seventeenth century merchants who risked their fortunes to finance long and dangerous sea voyages to distant parts of the world were the first to pool the risk of the loss of their vessels and cargo which would have meant bankruptcy. International commerce and business in general would be all but impossible without insurance. The welfare state might well be thought of as a large risk pool in which citizens participate to insure themselves against life's risks. Without the welfare state, a serious illness or the loss of a job could mean disaster for an individual family. Publicly funded health care, disability

R.J. Angel, J.L. Angel, *Hispanic Families at Risk*, DOI 10.1007/978-1-4419-0474-4_7,

and unemployment insurance, workers compensation, and the other programs of the welfare state ease the impact of such disasters.

A major problem related to the core theme of this book arises when the risk pool is not inclusive and leaves certain citizens to bear the burden of particular risks alone. The problem is compounded when exclusion from the risk pool is influenced by ascriptive characteristics such as race or ethnicity. Perhaps the insurance analogy seems a bit odd to those not used to thinking of social welfare programs in those terms, but the point is that certain groups, perhaps because of human capital deficits related to their group membership, are at risk of exclusion from basic social protections. As we have shown in the previous chapters, from birth to death Hispanic ethnicity places individuals at elevated risk, not only of low income and impaired social mobility but of increased vulnerability, inadequate medical care, and economic insecurity in old age. As we have also shown, Social Security and Medicare improve the situation of Hispanics after age 65, but public programs do little to address the vulnerabilities of working-age adults.

The Need for a Comprehensive Welfare State

We end this chapter with a general assessment of the welfare state in America and some observations concerning the possibilities for addressing the vulnerabilities we have identified in the Hispanic population. The issues we discuss apply to minority Americans generally, and even to poor non-Hispanic whites. To reiterate the observation with which we began, in an employment-based system of health and retirement benefits, those individuals and groups that are disadvantaged in the labor force are by definition disadvantaged in terms of economic security and health-care access throughout the life course and they face the serious risk of poverty in old age. The solution to this basic dilemma that the welfare state was introduced to deal with is to sever the tie between work and basic social rights. As we noted earlier, the modern welfare state was introduced by a conservative German government in the nineteenth century to deal with the social insecurities of a capitalist labor force. Capitalism, free markets, and the welfare state have been complementary developments. The welfare state protects capitalism from the inhumanities it generates that might lead workers to demand other arrangements. Yet debate over the extent and nature of the welfare state continues and the concept of social rights remains controversial.

Today, the United States faces the need to deal with holes in the social welfare safety net and problems with its incomplete welfare state. In all other developed nations, access to health care and other social rights is not dependent on employment as it is in the United States. The basis of the welfare state is moral as well as practical. In our opinion, in modern democracies social rights are as basic as political rights. Clearly, no nation can afford to provide everything citizens might want, but in a civilized nation access to the material basics of a dignified life cannot be sacrificed to budgetary considerations, especially when those material basics are inequitably distributed to begin with. Our greatest fear is that in the current economic crisis those who have never been incorporated into the economic and social mainstream may be further excluded. Peter Dwyer, speaking of the potential impact of the reduction of social benefits in Britain, notes that, even when justified on universal grounds, the reduction of benefits affects segments of the population selectively. The reduction of child benefits in Britain, for example, has a far more serious impact on poor single mothers than on middle-class couples (Dwyer 2004a).

Rather than basing our argument on the normative theoretical and ethical arguments related to the concept of social rights we have focused more on the practical outcomes of the exclusion of Hispanics for the material welfare of society as a whole. As we have argued throughout, one might view the poor, or at least a subset of the poor, as undeserving, but the reality is that given the low fertility and aging of the majority non-Hispanic white population, it will very soon find itself dependent on a minority labor force. The failure to attend to the education, health, and social needs of those groups means that the future labor force will be unable to and may well choose not to bear the economic burden of a population they see as hostile. Equity and normative morality aside, race and ethnicity continue to have very practical implications in the United States today.

Practical considerations and changing social and economic realities can and do result in organizational change where normative moral arguments do not. Historically, doctors, insurance companies, legislators, and even organized labor were opposed to universal health care, largely because of a profound distrust of government and a belief in the free market even in health care (Starr 1982). Today the rising cost of health coverage for average Americans, a growing population with no insurance, and the obvious waste brought about by an uncoordinated health-care system have changed almost everyone's mind (Daschle et al. 2008). The medical establishment, insurers, and the public in general are more receptive to the need to provide health-care coverage to everyone; the only question that remains is how. As the world becomes more complex and interdependent, the need for a functioning welfare state becomes clearer if a nation is to have a productive labor force and thrive in an increasingly challenging global economy (Esping-Andersen et al. 2002).

The core problem with health-care coverage, as with other aspects of the welfare state, arises from the fact that a voluntary employment-based or private health insurance system cannot, in principle, cover the entire population (Quaolagno, 2004). Unless coverage is mandatory, insurers will avoid what is termed "adverse risks," a term which refers to those individuals who need their services most. Individuals with preexisting conditions, people with mental illness, individuals with HIV/AIDS, and the poor generally are simply uninsurable. A profit-making or even nonprofit private enterprise cannot afford to incur the huge losses associated with providing care to individuals with multiple and expensive health-care needs. The only solution for a private insurer is to avoid individuals who are at elevated risk of poor health. In order to do so insurers engage in what is termed "underwriting," a term that refers to assessing each applicant for insurance to weed out the adverse risks (Gleeson 2004; Manton and Stallard 1992). Group insurance plans require the insurer to cover anyone who is hired by the company with at most some period of exclusion for preexisting conditions. Unemployed individuals or those who work for employers who do not offer a group plan are simply out of luck. Ideally, an equitable national health-care system would require that everyone be covered regardless of preexisting conditions, but that would inevitably require that medical risk be socialized, a concept that is anathema to many Americans. Our insurance analogy emphasizes the fact that unless we form a risk pool that includes all citizens our health-care system cannot be equitable. The same can be said for other basic social protections including income and housing. The poor, minorities, those with low-paying jobs, and those who represent adverse risks cannot be excluded without the denial of their basic social rights.

Minority Americans, including Hispanics, clearly benefit from Social Security, Medicare, Medicaid, and other means-tested programs for the poor. Yet, as we have shown, their levels of inclusion in the risk pool, especially for working-age adults are low. Initially Social Security did not cover agricultural or domestic workers, economic sectors that are heavily minority (Quadagno 1988a,b; Weir et al. 1988). In later years these workers and others were included in response to the growing acceptance of the proposition that no one should suffer the indignity of extreme poverty at the end of life. Until everyone is brought into the social risk pool, our social welfare state will remain incomplete and inequitable. As we continually note, this is unfair in and of itself, but it spells disaster for the nation's productivity in the future since a large fraction of the labor force is now and will be even more Hispanic and black in the very near future (Angel and Angel, 2006). The most basic economic stimulus program must be one that increases the productivity of these populations.

Framing the Problem: A More Effective Public Discourse

More than half a century after the most recent civil rights movement in the United States, race and ethnicity still influence the life chances of individuals, families, and communities. Clearly many important strides have been made toward equality in many domains. A half century ago African-Americans were unable to vote in many places; today we have our first African-American President. Yet for a large fraction of Americans, low levels of education, marginal employment, gangs, jail, and a life of blocked mobility are the realities of everyday life. Recent data from the Pew Hispanic Center reveal that between 1991 and 2007, the proportion of all federal prisoners who were Hispanic increased from 24% to 40%, largely because of increased enforcement of immigration laws (Lopez and Light 2009). These realities emerge from a complex history of exclusion, regional concentration, discrimination, and other factors unique to each group. The result is a lack of the material and social capital that other groups can call upon for education, to start businesses, and to help others in need.

The question that immediately comes to mind is why such large racial and ethnic disparities in everything from income to health-care coverage persist. With the removal of overtly discriminatory laws, one might have expected opportunity structures to have equalized, yet they have not. Mexican-origin students are not legally denied university admission, yet in 2005 while over a third of non-Hispanic white adults had a bachelor's degree or more, only 11.3% of Hispanics and only 8.3 of

Mexican-origin adults had earned a bachelor's degree or higher (National Center for Education Statistics 2007c). To characterize the problem, one might call upon the concept of "path dependence," a term used in political science and other disciplines to describe the inertia inherent in organizational structures (Pierson 2004). Once specific social structures and arrangements become institutionalized, they are very difficult to change. Those groups that benefit from the status quo, the winners, have little interest in altering the rules of the game and resist attempts to do so. But even those who do not necessarily benefit are constrained by tradition, established institutional arrangements, and habitual ways of interacting. Cultural institutions, such as the family and the church, socialize individuals into particular conceptions of social reality. Reference groups determine who one looks to as role models. If the available role models have little education, if they are unemployed or employed in low-wage jobs, and if they do not aspire to higher status, other than perhaps through crime, one has few examples of how to legitimately and effectively move ahead in life.

Conceptions of a culture of poverty have been offered to help explain how poverty and powerlessness become institutionalized and structure expectations and behaviors in ways that perpetuate poverty and powerlessness (Lewis 1959, 1966). Such explanations have been condemned for supposedly attributing mobility failure to something internal to the individual or his or her culture. Blaming the victim is clearly an unacceptable way of explaining poverty; the real objective should be to identify the structural and historical sources of disadvantage. Yet it would be a mistake to ignore the insidious and complex ways in which poverty harms individuals and the way it comes to pervade so much of social life (Wilson 2009). Powerlessness victimizes by undermining an individual's and a group's very ability to fight back, especially when powerlessness and poverty are accompanied by a stigmatized identity. The stigmatization of identity and the failure to recognize the inherent value of cultural differences represent a serious attack on individual autonomy and self-esteem (Fraser and Honneth 2003; Kymlicka 1995; Taylor 1994; Valadez 2001; Wilson 2009).

For the most part, the complexity of the sources of group-specific vulnerability is not part of a sophisticated public discourse. In the public mind, the issue of cultural diversity and multiculturalism, a term that has been introduced to refer to societies that include individuals from different backgrounds, is easily confounded with images of crime and street gangs, illegal immigration and drug smuggling, and much more that is negative. It is clear that the complexity of the tie between group membership, poverty, and the inability to escape poverty has not been successfully framed in public discourse in a way that convincingly focuses attention on the structural sources of the problems that certain groups face. For the most part, the failure of groups to move into the middle class is attributed to individual failure. We might ask how a more effective discourse might be introduced. Perhaps some comparison to the feminist movement would be useful, especially in terms of the relative success of feminism in framing the core problem of exclusion.

Women, or at least middle-class women, have been very effective in exposing the overt and covert structured sexism that affects the situation of women in almost all social institutions (Weinberg 2004). Fewer women than men make it to the higher tiers of business management; they are underrepresented among the leaders of major financial institutions; few reach flag rank in the military; and fewer women than men occupy prestigious endowed Chairs in the academy (Smith 2000). Yet the feminist movement has been very effective in framing the problem as one of endemic, structured, and pervasive sexism, rather than of individual failure. Major universities have responded by comprising committees to study the problem and in response to their recommendations have adopted procedures to address the core structural sources of gender-based inequity. This framing of the issues of differential power, exclusion, and the systematic preference given to the type of work that men perform is vital to defining the problem. Feminist academics have been very effective in pointing out that promotion committees, university procedures, and funding agencies are often biased in favor of the questions that men address and the methodological approaches they employ.

African-Americans and Hispanics have not been as successful in framing the problem of the almost complete lack of representation of minority faculty members in ways that result in effective remediation. Universities have certainly attempted diversity initiatives, but these have been more noble pronouncements than the clear commitment of resources to increase the number of minority faculty. Despite eloquent statements of institutional commitment to diversity, racial and ethnic representation on university faculties, and in other institutions, remains appallingly low. Attempts to redress the problem with real goals of increasing faculty and student representation are met with accusations of reverse discrimination. The problem of exclusion for minorities and the poor has not been framed in terms of a discourse that results in real action. In terms of framing the issues, African-Americans and Hispanics can clearly learn from feminists.

Unfortunately for minority Americans, the task of framing the discourse is confounded by the very structural problems that create the problem. While women are members of all social classes, including the highest, minority Americans are for the most part members of the lower classes where they have little contact with those in powerful positions and where they are less likely to attend the nation's most prestigeous universities. Without these opportunities they lack the contacts that might allow them to become members of networks with important business and political ties. While changing traditional sexist views is clearly difficult, the strategic location of highly articulate and effective spokeswomen is vitally important. Although there are clearly articulate and effective minority spokespersons, their access to power remains limited, and although the situation has clearly improved over the last several decades, minority groups still lack the material and social capital that might allow them to more effectively frame and widely communicate the discourse surrounding exclusion.

Framing a New Discourse of Inclusion

This new reality leads many social critics to question the ethnic and racial stratification that defines so much of modern life and to seek ways of reducing it. The core question is why certain groups still have little voice in public life or meaningful control over their lives even after decades of residence in the country. In Latin America and elsewhere, social critics are concerned with identifying the social requirements for active citizenship. This concept arises from the failure of the US-backed neoliberal market-based economic reforms of the 1980s and 1990s to address the serious inequities in income and access to vital social services in the region and to provide citizens the opportunity to participate in the decision-making processes concerning the organization of service delivery. Many parties, including the multilateral agencies that originally championed neoliberal reforms and a smaller role for government in the distribution of health and other services, have recognized the need to increase citizen and community involvement in the planning and administration of health care and other services (Chiara and Virgilio 2005; Tussie et al. 1997).

This new awareness of the need to empower citizens has accompanied the new interest in the role of civil society organizations, including churches, civic groups, political parties, and other nongovernmental organizations in giving citizens the power and knowledge to influence government and improve their own lives (Boli and Thomas 1997, 1999; Feinberg et al. 2006). Such attempts seek to give voice to previously voiceless peasants and poor communities. Unfortunately, the real ability of civil society organizations to further democratic objectives remains limited by the state and other actors (Shefner 2008). Nonetheless, the concept of active citizenship is central to our concerns in this book. The question we ask is why certain Hispanic groups remain outside of the economic and political mainstream even after generations. During the last two decades social theorists have begun to address the difficult social issues related to cultural and social group membership, identity, and social rights (Benhabib 2002; Fraser and Honneth 2003; Kymlicka 1995, 2007; Kymlicka and Norman 2000; Taylor 1994). Although we have focused more on practical issues rather than on normative moral arguments focused on equality, we must mention an important debate that is taking place in the academy. How one might apply the core moral points of that debate to address real-life inequities is worth thinking about.

The debate focuses on the moral basis for the coexistence of culturally and racially distinct groups so as to respect the culturally specific beliefs and practices of all. The objective is to provide some theoretical and practical insight into how different groups might live together equitably. The debate speaks to the core theme of this book since part of the problem of the exclusion of minority groups from the economic and social mainstreams results from their very different physiognomies and cultures. The utility of the multicultural debate is that it goes beyond the simple documentation of group disadvantage and focus on the normative dimensions of citizenship rights and the new multicultural political and social reality that confronts most nations of the world. The focus is on the rights and obligations of individuals from different racial and cultural groups, many of whom are immigrants, but some of whom are native and minority groups, who find themselves residents of the same nation state. The debate raises fundamental questions concerning the changing nature of the nation state system as well as the nature and function of civil society in defining rights and determining access to political and social power and influence.

Modern nation states are the result of long histories of group conflict, colonialism, internal displacement, and other processes that have resulted in often very culturally diverse populations occupying the same political region. The multicultural debate, therefore, is informed by a complex postcolonial politics and the recognition of important differences between colonized indigenous populations, refugees who have been forced to leave their homelands because of political unrest or natural disaster, and voluntary migrants who move in search of economic opportunities and political or religious freedom (Kymlicka 1995; Kymlicka and Norman 2000; Valadez 2001). While there is some acceptance of the proposition that the social and economic marginalization of colonized groups who were involuntary incorporated into nation states justifies some special treatment, often including the right to their own territory and the right to at least some degree of legal self-determination and special recognition of their cultural heritage, the situation of refugees, and certainly that of voluntary immigrants, is viewed differently. Individuals and groups who voluntarily leave their homelands and migrate to a new country are expected to assimilate rapidly and more completely, and they have fewer legitimate claims to special privileges. Voluntary immigrants are expected to learn the language and to adopt the host culture's mores and practices at least in public. Often they face proscriptions against the public display of aspects of their cultures of origin. As we noted in Chapter 2, the fact that new immigrants, and even long-time minority group residents, are ethnically and culturally very different creates serious problems for incorporation.

A well-publicized example from France occurred in 1989 when the Principal of the *collége Garriel-Havey* in Creil, France, expelled three Muslim girls for wearing the traditional Muslim scarf, the hijab, to school. The *foulard affair*, or scarf affair, as the incident came to be known, created much debate in France and elsewhere and raises issues that are as yet not resolved. France's official policy of *Laïcité*, which is often translated as "secularism," specifies that religious displays must be confined to the private realm (Poulat 2003). The policy is a response to the role of religion in public life in the past and is an attempt to insure that no belief system is granted special privileges. The foulard affair clearly reveals the difficulty western liberal democracies have with large ethnic and cultural differences. In an effort to maintain a strict separation between the state and religion, the acceptance of cultural differences can be difficult. In France, as in other countries in Europe, even when official policy emphasizes assimilation, voluntary migrants are often not allowed to fully incorporate into the host society and remain trapped in the legal and social limbo of a guest or temporary worker status, or that of illegal resident or undocumented alien.

Group Identity and Incorporation

The theme of immigration, then, brings us directly to the core of the problem of cultural diversity and tolerance in liberal welfare states as well as to the issue of the meaning of full social and economic participation. Today political debates in all receiving countries, including the nations of Western Europe and the United States, are dominated by loud calls for the control of borders and the enforcement of laws regarding illegal entry. Quieter debates that receive less media attention focus on the social and economic incorporation of those who have already arrived or of historically disadvantaged groups. In all countries one hears calls for mass deportations, but for the most part economic realities inform official governmental actions. Immigration and public policy must adapt to social and economic reality. Once individuals and families have arrived and established themselves, and even had children who have never known the country of origin, mass deportations are largely impossible. The more realistic response, in fact, is amnesty programs and policies that attempt at least to regularize and control the immigrant's situation. The simple reality is that modern industrial and globalized economies cannot function without cheap immigrant labor.

Cultural diversity, therefore, is assured and gives the cities of the developed world an increasingly international feel. Although many immigrants are highly educated and sought after for their technical skills and talents, many more, and especially those who cross frontiers illegally or overstay tourist visas, are less educated and do not qualify for special-skills visas. The result is that cultural diversity intersects systems of social and economic stratification, resulting in the overtly racial- and culture-based systems of inequality that we see today in Europe and elsewhere. The spatial and social marginalization of indigenous minorities and immigrant groups gives rise to demands for recognition of the basic worth of stigmatized cultures (Fraser and Honneth 2003; Kymlicka 1995; Kymlicka and Norman 2000; Taylor 1994). For multicultural theorists, one's culture of origin forms a central aspect of one's self-concept and the term "recognition" refers to the acceptance of the fundamental worth of one's cultural identity by others. Recognition also relates to one's racial and ethnic identity, especially when that is difficult to deny because of physical features. The alternative is stigmatization, a situation that undermines an individual's sense of self-worth and place in a society. In addition to recognition, theorists continue to argue for the need for redistribution, which refers to traditional concerns for the equitable distribution of material wealth (Fraser and Honneth 2003).

Both recognition and redistribution, though, are central to demands for social inclusion. While demands for recognition are based on the basic human need that one's personal and cultural identity be respected, such respect must also be accompanied by equity in access to material and political resources. The most serious danger that immigrants and indigenous minority populations face is exclusion from the means of economic and political power. The supportive and defensive civil society organizations that marginalized groups establish, including churches and professional associations, do not necessarily create ties to the larger culture or serve as avenues to political power. The basic problem arises from the fact that marginalized individuals and groups lack the ability to make their voices heard. Today, immigrants from Latin America do not become an active part of the municipal politics of the cities they inhabit in the same way that earlier immigrants did in nineteenth and early twentieth century Boston, Chicago, or New York. The marginalized situation of culturally distinct immigrants demands the conditions that proponents of communicative competence or deliberative democracy identify as ideal for the maximization of social rights (Ackerman and Fishkin 2004; Habermas 1984). Yet how these can be brought about remains unclear.

The long-term exclusion of individuals and groups from full participation in society has led theorists to ask what the basic requirements of involved or active citizenship are. While demographers and sociologists document the disadvantages that certain groups experience in terms of education, income, and social status, normative theorists deal with principled issues related to the requirements of a just and equitable society in which everyone participates fully regardless of their gender, race, ethnicity, or religious affiliation (Bessette 1994; Habermas 1984). Theoretical discussions of communicative rationality and deliberative democracy hold that true participation involves more than just voting, it requires the ability to engage in public discourse and requires a situation in which all participants have the capacity to engage in open and informed communication on an equal basis.

Such an ideal situation presupposes complete equality and, of necessity, equal access to power so it really represents the end to be achieved rather than the means to achieving that end. An individual cannot participate in conversation with even well-intentioned and liberal others without the capacity to educate himself and become a competent communicator. Achieving this status implies membership in a group that is either powerful historically or empowered by the state through such mechanisms as affirmative action programs, targeted investments, legislative quotas for stigmatized groups, or direct economic investment and support. Of course such support, even when well intentioned, can separate members of a group from the mainstream as in the case of indigenous populations that find themselves isolated on reservations.

Civil Society, Multiculturalism, and Active Citizenship

Several themes emerge in discussions of multiculturalism, immigration, and citizenship that are relevant to considerations of the situation of Hispanics in the United States. In the attempt to bring about situations in which the conditions for true participatory democracy exist, it is important to deal with issues of power and to examine the points of contact among immigrant groups and their ties, or lack of ties, to political parties and the political process generally. A major problem for the full economic and political incorporation of disadvantaged groups is their inability to engage in the machine politics that characterized the older immigration experiences of urban America. Self-help efforts do not necessarily translate into effective political movements and the failure to develop avenues to power poses serious problems for many Hispanic groups. An effective voice and the capacity for communicative competence require that the Hispanic population increase the number of its members with advanced degrees and the capacity to engage in effective communication. Such a critical mass could provide the role models that the community as a whole needs.

In addition, it is necessary to understand the role of institutions in empowering groups as a whole as well as their impact on individuals and communities. Within the framework of globalization and the international flow of labor, institutional theory provides the opportunity to examine the structural context within which migration occurs and in which certain groups remain marginalized. Identities and social connections, both of immigrants and of longer term citizens, are formed and maintained within political, religious, cultural, and legal institutions. Group identity and the reflexively created individual self do not exist in a vacuum, nor do they directly reflect beliefs, norms, practices, or symbolic systems of larger collectivities independent of their institutional context.

Culture inheres in institutions, as does political and economic power. Institutions provide opportunities for change at the same time that they constrain individual consciousness and freedom of action. For certain institutional theorists, institutions consist of the taken-for-granted rules of the game or the norms and belief systems that constrain individual actions. For others, institutions consist of the formal arrangements that define a corporate body or formally organized group enterprise. Recent work in institutional theory focuses on the role of ideas, in addition to interests, in determining institutional evolution (Campbell 2001; 2004; Ménard and Shirley 2005). Social institutions and their key actors help define and redefine social reality by providing cognitive frames in terms of which social actions are interpreted. Today, NGOs and other civil society institutions are part of the process of immigrant incorporation and also part of the attempt to change the image of the immigrant from that of dangerous foreigner to that of a productive addition to society. Their efforts to further a multicultural agenda are in direct opposition to the frames promoted by the far right. What is clear is that discussions of multiculturalism, incorporation, and cultural assimilation are dominated by interested and engaged institutions that embody and institutionalize various political perspectives. Understanding the role of such institutions in the process of migration is essential to understanding how structure and agency interact to determine the direction and content of cultural change as well as the degree of stigmatization or acceptance that immigrants experience.

The Central Role of Higher Education

Perhaps the most obvious mechanism through which structured disadvantage affects the Hispanic population, and the Mexican-origin population in particular, is the extremely low levels of education and high rates of school dropout that we have documented throughout the previous chapters (Romo and Falbo 1996; Telles and Ortiz 2008). Low educational levels and high dropout rates directly affect the probability of criminal activity and undermine one's employment and mobility chances. Low-wage work is unstable and does not allow the material and social capital accumulation that might result in significant group empowerment. Yet the extent of these disadvantages and their impact are not generally appreciated, or again they are viewed as simple individual failures rather than the outcomes of historically structured economic, social, and educational institutional arrangements. The apparent intractability of the problems of the Mexican-origin and African-American populations may in fact even have resulted in people turning off and not even paying attention to the causes or extent of those problems. Gangs, poor neighborhoods, crime, and poverty can be ignored if one does not find oneself in the midst of them, or again they can be viewed as individual or group failures.

Given their extremely low levels of education, it seems clear that Hispanic workers will continue to be overrepresented in the low-wage service sector. The limited productivity of this group will very soon become obvious and have serious collective impacts. The leading edge of the baby boom turned 62 in 2008 and in the immediate future the number of retirees receiving Social Security and Medicare will explode. In addition to bearing the burden of a growing retired population, working-age Americans will have to deal with the massive deficits required for the stimulus packages intended to jump start the economy after the recession of 2008. They will have to assume the risk of bailing out the auto industry. They will pay for the massive military presence in Afghanistan and the rest of the covert war on terrorism, and much more. The labor force of the future may be simply unable to bear the burden no matter what. If, as we have continually noted, a large fraction of that labor force is Hispanic and has low levels of productivity, the economic failure of the system is almost assured. The only recourse will be a massive decrease in everyone's standard of living and a retreat by the United States from its more expensive and ambitious international commitments.

Perhaps the most obvious approach to addressing the problem of low educational levels and high dropout rates among Hispanics is to focus on increasing their retention rates in high school and improving their educational performance. We clearly agree with those objectives and every effort should be made to bring them about. The core problem has been that despite our best efforts, dropout rates remain extremely high and school performance low. While strongly supporting the focus on primary and secondary school retention and performance, we propose a different approach to the problem of educational deficits in the Hispanic population. Our proposal is to focus aggressively on increasing the number of Hispanics with baccalaureate and post-graduate degrees who might serve as role models and advocates for the group as a whole.

Education, and especially post-secondary education, not only provides one with general and specific knowledge and skills, but it inculcates and reinforces middle-class values, specifically those related to occupational and social mobility. Each morning middle-class children see their parents dress for work, leave at a specified hour, and return on schedule at the end of the day. In middle-class neighborhoods these children see their friends' parents do the same. These children are aware that their parents earn salaries that allow the family to live a middle-class lifestyle and enjoy the material benefits that all families desire. In such a situation children see clear examples of how education, hard work, and the routine of a career can pay off in high-quality lives. That socialization is often so effective that children become overachievers themselves and in primary and secondary schools already find themselves in a race to excel.

In poor neighborhoods the situation is completely different. Clearly, many low-income families are highly functional and many poor neighborhoods have strong neighborhood ties and significant social capital. As statistics on crime rates, gang activity, family disruption, transience, and other negative social indictors clearly show, though, many poor neighborhoods are hardly ideal places in which to grow up. Unlike middle-class neighborhoods in which the value of education and regular employment is clear, in many poor neighborhoods children do not see their parents engaged in routines based on well-paying jobs with benefits, nor do they see their friends' parents enjoying the benefits of careers. In such neighborhoods unemployment is high and many parents, and especially single parents, work primarily in low-wage and irregular jobs. Food stamps, welfare, and the other markers of insecurity are common. Children in these neighborhoods do not grow up with the examples of the connection between educational achievement and material rewards that middle-class children grow up with. Rather, they often see that criminal and gang activity is what is rewarded materially and socially.

This observation leads us to suggest that perhaps the most realistic and immediate way to address the problem of low educational levels and the lack of access to powerful positions for the community as a whole is to focus much more time and effort on higher education. The first instinct of social progressives, and indeed one legitimate way of viewing the educational problem, is to focus on primary and secondary education. Clearly, if a young person drops out of school in the ninth grade and never returns, he or she is in no position to go on to higher education and to a profession. Viewing the situation as a "pipeline" problem in which there are too few individuals successfully completing the most basic levels of education to result in substantial numbers entering university is clearly rational. Yet it is difficult to deny that we have had limited success in addressing the problems of dropping out and low performance in secondary education.

In light of our discussion of the middle-class nature of education, we suggest that it may make sense to address the problem of the lack of positive educational role models by aggressively increasing the number of Hispanic individuals with bachelor's and post-graduate degrees and the number of Hispanic faculty members in American universities. Even if these individuals do not become advocates, by their very presence they can change perceptions. If a quarter of the faculty of a university or law school, or a fifth of the doctors in a prestigious medical practice had Spanish surnames, young people would have clear evidence that education pays off. Today, faculty members with Spanish surnames are rare. Unlike attempts to increase retention in secondary school which requires addressing multiple complex social problems, increasing the number of students in graduate and professional schools and on university faculties can be done more directly. Admissions and hiring practices can be examined to reveal systematic barriers to inclusion. If only the students of professors well known to faculty members are interviewed and hired, or if certain theoretical or methodological approaches are given more weight because those are familiar to evaluators, few minority group faculty will be hired. Feminists have clearly pointed out this problem in the case of female faculty representation. The frequently made claim that minority faculty members are simply not available is suspect in our view. As is the case with women, an effective discourse on the situation of Hispanic and minority representation at the higher levels of institutional management is necessary.

While focusing on structural barriers to higher levels of Hispanic and minority inclusion in middle-class life, we must also recognize the responsibility the Hispanic community itself has in promoting its own interests and that of its children and grandchildren. Educational opportunities are useless unless they are taken advantage of. Successful middle-class students take advance placement courses and pursue clearly competitive curricula because their parents have high expectations for them. Students whose parents show little interest in their education or their eventual success are far less likely to do the same. Welfare reform in the United States and the new third way in Europe that we discussed earlier emphasize that there are no rights without duties. While such claims can be used as a justification for denying poor individuals basic services, they clearly reflect a public expectation that individuals should help themselves. At the same time that we increase the number of Hispanic professionals with higher levels of education, they and the community at large must recognize the collective obligation to support the most promising students in their effort to go to college and beyond. Hispanic parents must become more interested in their children's daily educational activities. They should also accept the fact that their children often must move away from home and the community to attend the best colleges and universities. These changes require community outreach and communication programs that inform parents and their children of the opportunities for admission and funding that exist at the nation's top universities. Until the community has a substantial number of successful role models, though, such efforts will be difficult to implement.

Individual and Group Mobility, the Welfare State, and the American Future

We end then with a reaffirmation of the welfare state both on principled moral grounds and on very practical grounds. Clearly, everyone should take as much responsibility for their own welfare as possible. Yet as human history clearly shows, complete self-sufficiency is not part of the human situation. We spent most of our history in tribes and completely interdependent on one another for the basics of life. To be ostracized from the tribe was to be condemned to near certain death. Today, serious physical illness, economic collapse, epidemic disease, and much more reveal our ultimate interdependence. Even the most supposedly self-sufficient among us is dependent on the welfare state for health care, retirement income, education, and more. Capitalism and the welfare state are mutually supporting and make our modern world possible. The recession of 2008 clearly revealed the vulnerability of everyone to economic downturns and the fact that for the weak and vulnerable such downturns are devastating.

As we hopefully have demonstrated, the vulnerabilities of the Hispanic population reveal many of the inherent weaknesses of the employment-based social welfare system in insuring not only individual well-being but also the future survivability of our collective economic and social enterprise. The academic discussions of multiculturalism and social rights we have briefly touched upon focus on the inherent fairness of the social arrangements that one might ideally desire and the contrast between those ideals and the historical reality that determines where in the social and economic hierarchy individuals and groups find themselves. The harsh reality of life is that individuals and groups are in competition for scarce resources, including the best jobs and admission to prestigious colleges and universities. Today, affirmative action and other direct attempts to increase minority representation in university admissions and on faculties, as well as in other domains in which they remain underrepresented, are met with strong resistance. The relatively short-term negative consequences of such exclusion for everyone, though, must be made clear to the American public. As we have argued, the long-term consequences of such structured exclusion will be disastrous for the nation. The most important mid- and long-term economic stimulus that we can suggest is a major investment in the higher education of the nation's Hispanic and minority populations.

References

Achenbaum W. Andrew. 1986. *Social Security: Visions and Revisions.* New York: Cambridge University Press.

Ackerman, Bruce, and James S. Fishkin. 2004. *Deliberation Day.* New Haven, CT: Yale University Press.

Agency for Healthcare Research and Quality. 2005. *Employer-Sponsored Health Insurance: Trends in Cost and Access.* Washington, DC: Agency for Healthcare Research and Quality.

Alamo Area Council of Governments. 2007. *Bexar County Area Plan: Fiscal Years 2008–2010.* San Antonio, TX: Area Agency on Aging.

Alba, Richard D. 1990. *Ethnic Identity: The Transformation of White America.* New Haven, CN: Yale University Press.

Alba, Richard D., and Victor Nee. 2003. *Remaking the American Mainstream: Assimilation and the New Immigration*: Cambridge, MA: Harvard University Press.

Amey, Cheryl, Karen Seccombe, and R. Paul Duncan. 1995. "The Health Insurance Coverage of Mexican-American Families in the United States: The Effect of Employment Context and Family Structure in Rural and Urban Settings." *Journal of Family Issues* 16:488–510.

Anderson, Steven G., and Mary Keegan Eamon. 2004. "Health Coverage Instability for Mothers in Working Families." *Social Work* 49:395–405.

Angel, Jacqueline L. 2003. "Devolution and the Social Welfare of Elderly Immigrants: Who Will Bear the Burden?" *Public Administration Review* 63:79–89.

Angel, Jacqueline L., Ronald J. Angel, Maria P. Aranda, and Toni P. Miles. 2004. "Can the Family Still Cope? Social Support and Health as Determinants of Nursing Home Use in the Older Mexican-origin Population." *Journal of Aging and Health* 16:338–354.

Angel, Jacqueline L., and Dennis P. Hogan. 2004. "Population Aging and Diversity in a New Era." pp. 128–139 in *Closing the Gap: Improving the Health of Minority Elders in the New Millennium*, edited by Keith E. Whitfield. Washington, DC: Gerontological Society of America.

Angel, Jacqueline L., and Keith E. Whitfield (Eds.). 2007. *The Health of Aging Hispanics: The Mexican-Origin Population.* New York: Springer.

Angel, Ronald, and Laura Lein. 2006. "The Myth of Self-Sufficiency in Health." pp. 99–112 in *Women, Working and Welfare in San Antonio*, edited by Jane Henrici. Tucon, AZ: University of Arizona Press.

Angel, Ronald J., and Jacqueline L. Angel. 1996. "The Extent of Private and Public Health Insurance Coverage Among Adult Hispanics." *The Gerontologist* 36:332–340.

Angel, Ronald J., and Jacqueline L. Angel. 1997. *Who Will Care For Us? Aging and Long-Term Care in Multicultural America.* New York: New York University Press.

Angel, Ronald J., and Jacqueline L. Angel. 2006. "Aging and Diversity." pp. 94–110 in *Handbook of Aging and the Social Sciences*, edited by Robert Binstock and Linda George. San Diego, CA: Academic.

Angel, Ronald J., and Jacqueline L. Angel. 2007. "The Health Care Safety Net for Hispanics." pp. 263–279 in *The Health of Aging Hispanics: The Mexican-Origin Population*, edited by Jacqueline L. Angel and Keith E. Whitfield. New York: Springer.

Angel, Roand J., Jacqueline L. Angel, and Kyriakos S. Markides. 2002. "Stability and Change in Health Insurance Among Older Mexican Americans: Longitudinal Evidence from the Hispanic Established Populations for Epidemiologic Study of the Elderly." *American Journal of Public Health* 92:1264–1271.

Angel, Ronald J., Jacqueline L. Angel, and Jennifer K. Montez. 2009. "The Work/Health Insurance Nexus: A Weak Link for Mexican-origin Men." *Social Science Quarterly* 90(x).

Angel, Ronald J., Jacqueline L. Angel, and Laura Lein. 2007. "The Health Care Safety Net for Mexican American Families." pp. 395–410 in *Handbook of Families and Poverty*, edited by D. Russell Crane and Tim B. Heaton. Thousand Oaks, CA: Sage Publications.

Angel, Ronald J., Laura Lein, and Jane Henrici. 2006. *Poor Families in America's Health Care Crisis*. New York: Cambridge University Press.

Asher, Robert, and Charles Stephenson (Eds.). 1990. *Labor Divided : Race and Ethnicity in United States Labor Struggles, 1835–1960*. Albany, N.Y.: State University of New York Press.

Atherly, Adam, and Kenneth E. Thorpe. 2005. *Value of Medicare Advantage to Low-Income and Minority Medicare Beneficiaries*. Atlanta, GA: Rollins School of Public Health, Emory University.

Baker, Susan Gonzalez. 1999. "Mexican-Origin Women in Southwestern Labor Markets." pp. 244–269 in *Latinas and African American Women at Work: Race, Gender, and Economic Inequality*, edited by Irene Browne. New York: Russell Sage Foundation.

Balibar, Étienne. 2004. We, The People of Europe? *Reflections on Transnational Citizenship*. Princeton, NJ: Princeton University Press.

Bean, Frank D., and Stephanie Bell-Rose. 1999. *Immigration and Opportunity: Race, Ethnicity, and Employment in the United States*. New York: Russell Sage Foundation.

Bean, Frank D., and Marta Tienda. 1990. *The Hispanic Population of the United States*. New York: Russell Sage Foundation.

Bengtson, Vern L., and W. A. Achenbaum. 1993. *The Changing Contract Across Generations*. New York: Aldine.

Benhabib, Seyla. 2002. *The Claims of Culture: Equality and Diversity in the Global Era*. Princeton, NJ: Princeton University Press.

Berkowitz, Edward D. 1991. *America's Welfare State: From Roosevelt to Reagan* Baltimore, MD: Johns Hopkins University.

Bernstein, Amy B., Robin A. Cohen, Kate M. Brett, and Mary A. Bush. 2008. *Marital Status is Associated with Health Insurance Coverage for Working-Age Women at All Income Levels: 2007*. Hyattsville, MD: National Center for Health Statistics.

Bessette, Joseph M. 1994. *The Mild Voice of Reason: Deliberative Democracy and American National Government*. Chicago: University of Chicago Press.

Boli, John, and George M. Thomas. 1997. "World Culture in the World Polity: A Century of International Non-Governmental Organization." *American Sociological Review* 62:171–190.

Boli, John, and George M. Thomas (Eds.). 1999. *Constructing World Culture: International Non-Governmental Organizations Since 1875*. Stanford, CA: Stanford University Press.

Bongaarts, John. 2004. "Population Aging and the Rising Cost of Public Pensions." in *Working Paper*, edited by Policy Research Division. New York and Washington, DC: Population Council.

Borjas, George. 1985. "Jobs and Employment for Hispanics." pp. 144–157 in *Hispanics in the United States: A New Social Agenda*, edited by Pastora Cafferty and William C. McCready. New Brunswick, NJ: Transaction Publisher.

Borjas, George, and Lawrence F. Katz. 2007. *The Evolution of the Mexican-Born Workforce in the United States*. pp. 13–55. Cambridge, MA: National Bureau of Economic Research.

Borjas, George J. 1990. *Friends or Strangers: The Impact of Immigrants on the U.S. Economy*. New York: Basic Books.

Braithwaite, John. 2005. "Inequality and Republican Criminology." pp. 277–305 in *Crime and Inequality*, edited by John Hagan and Ruth D. Peterson. Palo Alto, CA: Stanford University.

Broaddus, Matthew, and Leighton Ku. 2000. *Nearly 95 Percent of Low-Income Uninsured Children Now Are Eligible for MEDICAID or SCHIP: Measures Need to Increase Enrollment Among Eligible But Uninsured Children*. Washington, D.C.: Center on Budget and Policy Priorities.

Bureau of Labor Statistics. 2001. *How the Government Measures Unemployment*. Washington, DC: Bureau of Labor Statistics, Division of Labor Force Statistics.

Bureau of Labor Statistics. 2003. *Differences in Women's and Men's Earnings by Race and Hispanic Origin*. Washington, DC: U.S. Department of Labor.

Bureau of Labor Statistics. 2008. *Employment Status by Hispanic Ethnicity and Detailed Ethnic Group*. Washington, DC: Bureau of Labor Statistics.

Bureau of Labor Statistics. 2009a. *The Employment Situation: January 2009*. Washington, DC: U.S. Department of Labor.

Bureau of Labor Statistics. 2009b. *Employment Status of the Hispanic or Latino Population by Sex and Age*. Washington, DC: U.S. Department of Labor.

Bureau of Labor Statistics. 2009c. *Union Affiliation of Employed Wage and Salary Workers by Selected Characteristics: 2008*. Washington, DC: U.S. Department of Labor.

Campbell, John L. 2004. *Institutional Change and Globalization*. Princeton, NJ: Princeton University Press.

Campbell, John L., and Ove K. Pedersen (Eds.). 2001. *The Rise of Neoliberalism and Institutional Analysis*. Princeton, NJ: Princeton University Press.

Carliner, David. 2002. "Getting the Elderly Their Due." *Health Affairs* 21:198–201.

Casteles, Stephen. 2004. "Why Migration Policies Fail." *Ethnic and Racial Studies* 27:205–227.

Catanzarite, Lisa, and Vilma Ortiz. 2002. "Too Few Good Men? Available Partners and Single Motherhood Among Latinas, African Americans, and Whites." *Hispanic Journal of Behavioral Sciences* 24:278–295.

Center for American Progress. 2004. *How Social Security Benefits the Latino Community*. Washington, DC: Center for American Progress.

Centers for Medicare and Medicaid Services. 1999. *The State Children's Health Insurance Program Annual Enrollment Report: October 1, 1998 to September 30, 1999*. Baltimore, MD: Centers for Medicare and Medicaid Services.

Centers for Medicare and Medicaid Services. 2005. *State Children's Health Insurance Program Summary*. Baltimore, MD: Centers for Medicare and Medicaid Services.

Centers for Medicare and Medicaid Services. 2008. "Who is Eligible for Medicare." *in Medicare Eligibility Tool*. Washington, DC: U.S. Department of Health and Human Services.

Chiara, Magdalena, and Mercedes di Virgilio. 2005. *Gestión Social y Municipios. De los escritorios del Banco Mundial a los barrios del Gran Buenos Aires*. Buenos Aires, Argentina: Prometeo Libros-UNGS.

Child Trends. 2005. *High School Dropout Rates*. Washington, DC: Child Trends Data Bank.

Child Trends Data Bank. 2003. *Health Care Coverage*. Washington, DC: Child Trends Data Bank.

Children's Defense Fund. 2006. *Improving Children's Health: Understanding Children's Health Disparities and Promising Approaches to Address Them*. Washington, DC: Children's Defense Fund.

Chollet, Deborah. 1994. "Employer-Based Health Insurance in a Changing Work Force." *Health Affairs* 13:315–326.

Congressional Budget Office. 2007. *State Children's Health Insurance Program*. Washington, DC: Congress of the United States.

Coontz, Stephanie. 2000. *The Way We Never Were: American Families and the Nostalgia Trap*. New York: Basic Books.

Copeland, Craig. 2005. "Employment-Based Retirement Plan Participation: Geographic Differences and Trends, 2004" in *Issues Brief*. Washington, DC: Employment Benefit Research Institute.

Copeland, Craig. 2007. *Employment-Based Retirement Plan Participation: Geographic Differences and Trends, 2006*. Washington, DC: Employment Benefit Research Institute.

Crosnoe, Robert. 2006. *Mexican Roots, American Schools: Helping Mexican Immigrant Children Succeed*. Palo Alto, CA: Stanford University Press.

Crystal, Stephen. 1982. *America's Old Age Crisis*. New York: Basic Books.

Current Population Survey. 2004–06. *2006 Annual Social and Economic (ASEC) Supplement*. Washington, DC: U.S. Census Bureau, Government Printing Office.

Current Population Survey. 2006. *Employed Persons by Occupation, Race, Hispanic or Latino Ethnicity and Sex*. Washington, DC: U.S. Department of Labor, U.S. Bureau of the Census.

Current Population Survey. 2008a. *POV 10, People in Families by Number of Working Family Members and Family Structure: 2007*. Washington, DC: U.S. Bureau of the Census.

Daschle, Tom, Jeanne M. Lambrew, and Scott S. Greenberger. 2008. *Critical: What We Can Do about the Health-Care Crisis*. New York: MacMillan Books.

de la Garza, Rodolfo O. 2005. "Latino Immigrants, National Identity and the National Interest." in *The Baby Bust: Who Will Do the Work? Who Will Pay the Taxes?* Washington, DC: Eisenhower Foundation.

DeNavas-Walt, Carmen, Bernadette D. Proctor, and Jessica C. Smith. 2008. *Income, Poverty, and Health Insurance Coverage in the United States: 2007*. Washington DC: U.S. Census Bureau.

Dorn, Stan, Bowen Garrett, John Holahan, Aimee Williams, and Kaiser Permanente. 2009. *Medicaid, SCHIP and Economic Downturn: Policy Challenges and Policy Responses*. Menlo Park, CA: The Henry J. Kaiser Family Foundation.

Dubay, Lisa, Jennifer M. Haley, and Genevieve M. Kenney. 2002. "Children's Eligibility for Medicaid and SCHIP: A View from 2000." in *New Federalism: National Survey of America's Families*. Washington, DC: Urban Institute.

Duncan, Brian, V. Joseph Hotz, and Stephen J. Trejo. 2006. "Hispanics in the U.S. Labor Market." pp. 228–290 in *Hispanics and the Future of America*, edited by Marta Tienda and Faith Mitchell. Washington, DC: The National Academies Press.

Duncan, Brian, and Steven J. Trejo. 2005. "Ethnic Identification, Intermarriage, and Unmeasured Progress by Mexican Americans." in *Working Papers* 11423. Washington, DC: National Bureau of Economic Research.

Dwyer, Peter. 2004a. "Creeping Conditionality in the UK: From Welfare Rights to Conditional Entitlements?" *The Candaian Journal of Sociology* 29:265–287.

Dwyer, Peter. 2004b. *Understanding Social Citizenship*. Bristol, England: The Policy Press and the Social Policy Association.

East, Patricia L. 1998. "Racial and Ethnic Differences in Girls' Sexual, Marital, and Birth Expectations." *Journal of Marriage and Family* 60:150–162.

Eichner, June, and Bruce C. Vladeck. 2005. "Medicare as a Catalyst for Reducing Health Disparities." *Health Affairs* 24:365–375.

Eisert, Sheri, and Patricia Gabow. 2002. "Effect of Child Health Insurance Plan Enrollment on the Utilization of Health Care Services by Children Using a Public Safety Net System." *Pediatrics* 110:940–945.

Eldridge, Gloria Nicole. 2007. "The Medicaid Evolution: The Political Economy of Medicaid Federalism." in *Doctoral Dissertation*. Austin, TX: The University of Texas at Austin.

Employee Benefit Research Institute. 2005. *Fundamentals of Employee Benefit Programs*. Washington, DC: Employee Benefit Research Institute.

Employee Benefits Research Institute. 2008. "Retirement Annuity and Employment-Based Pension Income Among Individuals Age 50 and Over: 2007." *Notes* 29:1–10.

Engelhardt, Gary V., and Jonathan Gruber. 2004. "Social Security and the Evolution of Elderly Poverty." in *NBER Working Paper Series*. Cambridge, MA: National Bureau of Economic Research.

Escarce, José J., and Kanika Kapur. 2006. "The Health Status and Health Behaviors of Hispanics." pp. 410–446 in *Hispanics and the Future of America*, edited by Marta Tienda and Faith Mitchell. Washington, DC: National Academy Press.

Eschbach, Karl, Soham Al-Snih, Kyriakos S. Markides, and James S. Goodwin. 2007. "Disability and Active Life Expectancy of Older U.S.- and Foreign Born Mexican Americans." pp. 40–49 in *The Health of Aging Hispanics: The Mexican-Origin Population*, edited by Jacqueline L. Angel and Keith E. Whitfield. New York: Springer.

Esping-Andersen, Gøsta. 1990. *The Three Worlds of Welfare Capitalism*. Princeton, NJ: Princeton University Press.

Esping-Andersen, Gøsta. 1999. *Social Foundations of Postindustrial Economies*. Oxford; New York: Oxford University Press.

Esping-Andersen, Gøsta, Duncan Gallie, Anton Hemerijck, and John Myles. 2002. *Why We Need A New Welfare State*. New York: Oxford University Press.

Espinosa, Ruben, and Alberto Ochoa. 1986. "Concentration of California Hispanic Students in Schools with Low Achievement: A Research Note." *American Journal of Education* 95:77–95.

Etzioni, Amitai. 1993. *The Spirit of Community: Rights, Responsibilities, and the Communitarian Agenda*. New York: Crown Publishers.

Etzioni, Amitai (Ed.). 1995. *New Communitarian Thinking: Persons, Virtues, Institutions, and Communities*. Charlottesville: Virginia University Press of Virginia.

Etzioni, Amitai. 2000. *The Third Way to a Good Society*. London: Demos.

Everett, Bethany G., Richard G. Rogers, Patrick M. Krueger, and Robert A. Hummer. 2007. "Trends in Educational Attainment by Sex, Race/Ethnicity, and Nativity in the United States: 1989–2005." University of Colorado Population Program Working Paper #2007–07.

Federal Interagency Forum on Aging-Related Statistics. 2008. "Older Americans Update 2008: Key Indicators of Well-Being." edited by National Center for Health Statistics. Washington, DC: U.S. Government Printing Office.

Feinberg, Richard, Carlos H. Waisman, and Leon Zamosc (Eds.). 2006. *Civil Society and Democracy in Latin America*. New York: Pelgrave MacMillan.

Finkle, Tori, Heidi Hartmann, and Sunhwa Lee. 2007. "Economic Security Among Older People in the United States: Gender and Race/Ethnic Disparities Persist." pp. Table 2 in *Briefing Paper Series*. Washington, DC: Institute for Women's Policy Research.

Flippen, Chenoa, and Marta Tienda. 2000. "Pathways to Retirement: Patterns of Labor Force Participation and Labor Market Exit Among the Pre-Retirement Population by Race, Hispanic Origin, and Sex." *Journal of Gerontology: Social Sciences* 55:S14–S27.

Flynn, Don. 2005. "New Borders, New Management: The Dilemmas of Modern Immigration Policies." *Ethnic and Racial Studies* 28:463–490.

Fraser, Nancy, and Alex Honneth. 2003. *Redistribution or Recognition? A Political-Philosophical Exchange*. New York: Verso.

Frey, William H. 2006. *Diversity Spreads Out: Metropolitan Shifts in Hispanic, Asian, and Black Populations Since 2000*. Washington, DC: Brookings Institution.

Fronstin, Paul. 2005a. "The Relationship Between Income and Health Insurance: Rethinking the Use of Family Income in the Current Population Survey." in *EBRI Notes*. Washington, DC: Employee Benefit Research Institute.

Fronstin, Paul. 2005b. "Sources of Health Insurance and Characteristics of the Uninsured: Analysis of the March 2005 Current Population Survey." Washington, DC: Employee Benefit Research Institute.

Fry, Richard, Rakesh Kochhar, Jeffrey Passel, and Roberto Suro. 2005. "Hispanics and the Social Security Debate." Washington, DC: Pew Hispanic Center Project.

Gans, Herbert J. 1992. "Comment: Ethnic Invention and Acculturation: A Bumpy-Line Approach." *Journal of American Ethnic History* 11:42–52.

Gassoumis, Zachary D., Kathleen H. Wilber, and Fernando Torres-Gil. 2008. "Latino Baby Boomers: A Hidden Population." pp. 1–4 in *Latinos and Social Security*. Los Angeles, CA: University of California Los Angeles; Center for Policy Research on Aging.

Giddens, Anthony. 1998. *The Third Way: The Renewal of Social Democracy*. Malden, MA: Blackwell Publishers Inc.

Gilbert, Neil, and Barbara Gilbert. 1989. *The Enabling State: Modern Welfare Capitalism in America*. Oxford, Eng.: Oxford University Press.

Gleeson, Robert K. 2004. "Medical Underwriting." pp. 73–94 in *Genetics and Life Insurance: Medical Underwriting and Social Policy*, edited by Mark A. Rothstein. Cambridge, MA: Massachussetts Institute of Technology Press.

Gordon, Milton M. 1964. *Assimilation in American Life: The Role of Race, Religion, and National Origins*. New York: Oxford University Press.

Gottschalk, Marie. 2000. *The Shadow Welfare State: Labor, Business, and the Politics of Health-Care in the United States*. Ithaca, NY: ILR Press.

Greenwald, Matthew. 2007. "The Rockefeller Foundation, Minority Retirement Confidence Survey." Washington, DC: Employee Benefit Research Institute.

Grossman, Brian R., Erica Solway, Brooke A. Hollister, Carroll L. Estes, and Leah Rogne. 2008. "One Nation, Interdependent: Exploring the Boundaries of Citizenship in the History of Social Security and Medicare." pp. 115–147 in *Social Insurance and Social Justice,* edited by Leah Rogne, Carroll L. Estes, Brian R. Grossman, Brooke A. Hollister, and Erica Solway. New York: Springer Publishing Company.

Gurewich, Deborah, Jeffrey Prottas, Robert Seifert, and Susan Seager. 2004. "Medical Debt and Consumer Credit Counseling Services." *Journal of Health Care for the Poor and Underserved* 15:336–346.

Guyer, Jocelyn. 2000. *Health Care after Welfare: An Update of Findings from State-Level Leaver Studies*. Washington, DC: Center for Budget and Policy Priorities.

Habermas, Jurgen. 1984. *The Theory of Communicative Action*, Vol. 1. Boston: Beacon Press.

Hacker, Jacob S. 2002. *The Divided Welfare State*. New York: Cambridge University Press.

Hagan, John, and Ruth Peterson. 1995. "Criminal Inequality in America: Patterns and Consequences." pp. 14–36 in *Crime and Inequality* edited by John Hagan and Ruth D. Peterson. Palo Alto, CA: Stanford University Press.

Hahn, Beth A. 1993. "Marital Status and Women's Health: The Effect of Economic Marital Acquisitions." *Journal of Marriage and Family* 55:495–504.

Ham-Chande, Roberto. 2008. *Economic Sustainability of Retirement Pensions in Mexico: Is There a Link with the Mexican-Origin Population in the United States?* Orlando, FL: Society of Actuaries.

Hamilton, Erin R., Robert A. Hummer, Xiuhong H. You, and Yolanda C. Padilla. 2006. "Health Insurance and Health-Care Utilization of U.S.-Born Mexican-American Children." *Social Science Quarterly* 87:1280–1294.

Hayes-Bautista, David E. 2004. *La Nueva California: Latinos and California Society, 1940–2040.* Berkeley, CA: The University of California Press.

He, Wan. 2002. "The Older Born Foreign-Born Population in the United States: 2000." in *Current Population Reports* p 23–211. Washington, DC: U.S. Bureau of the Census.

Heinz, Walter R. 2004. "From Work Trajectories to Negotiated Careers. The Contingent Work Life Course." pp. 185–204 in *Handbook of the Life Course,* edited by Jeylan T. Mortimer and Michael J. Shanahan. New York, Springer.

Helman, Ruth, Matthew Greenwald, Jack VanDerhei, and Craig Copeland. 2007. *Minority Workers Remain Confident About Retirement, Despite Lagging Preparations and False Expectations.* Washington, DC: Employee Benefit Research Institute.

Hendley, Alexa A., and Natasha F. Bilimoria. 1999. *Minorities and Social Security: An Analysis of Racial and Ethnic Differences in the Current Program.* Baltimore, MD: Office of Retirement Policy, Office of Policy, Social Security Administration.

Herd, Pamela. 2005. "Reforming a Breadwinner Welfare State: Gender, Race, Class and Social Security Reform." *Social Forces* 83:1365–1393.

Hicks, Alexander. 1999. *Social Democracy and Welfare Capitalism.* Ithaca, NY: Cornell University Press.

Higginbotham, Elizabeth. 1997. "Introduction." pp. xv–xxxii in *Women and Work. Exploring Race, Ethnicity, and Class,* edited by Elizabeth Higginbotham and Mary Romero. Thousand Oaks, CA: Sage Publications, Inc.

Himmelstein, David U., Elizabeth Warren, Deborah Thorne, and Steffie Woolhandler. 2005. "Market Watch: Illness and Injury as Contributors to Bankruptcy." in *Health Affairs- Web Exclusive, February 2*.

Hirsch, Barry T., David A. MacPherson, and J. Michael Dumond. 1997. "Workers' Compensation Recipiency in Union and Nonunion Workplaces." *Industrial and Labor Relations Review* 50:213–236.

Holley, Hana. 2006. "Retirement Planning Survey Among Hispanic U.S. Adults Age 40 and Older: Executive Summary." in *Strategic Issues Research, AARP*. Washington, DC: AARP.

Holt, Steve. 2006. "The Earned Income Tax Credit at Thirty: What We Know." in *The Metropolitan Policy Program*. Washington, DC: The Brookings Institution.

Hondagneu-Sotelo, Pierrette. 1997. "Working 'Without Papers' in the United States." pp. 101–125 in *Women and Work. Exploring Race, Ethnicity, and Class,* edited by Elizabeth Higginbotham and Mary Romero. Thousand Oaks, CA: Sage Publications, Inc.

Hondagneu-Sotelo, Pierrette. 2001. *Doméstica: Immigrant Workers Cleaning and Caring in the Shadows of Influence*. Los Angeles, CA: University of California Los Angeles.

Hounsell, Cindy, Anna Rappaport, Jeff Lewis, and Alison Kane. 2006. *Unique Challenges Faced by Women in Preparing for and Managing Their Retirement Years*. Washington, DC: Women's Institute for a Secure Retirement.

Howard, Chrstopher. 1997. *The Hidden Welfare State: Tax Expenditures and Social Policy in the United States*. Princeton, NJ: Princeton University Press.

Huntington, Samuel P. 2004. "The Hispanic Challenge." *Foreign Policy* Mar/Apr:30–45.

Huynh, Phuong Trang, Cathy Schoen, Robin Osborn, and Alyssa L. Holmgren. 2006. *The U.S. Health Care Divide: Disparities in Primary Care Experiences by Income*. New York: The Commonwealth Fund.

Institute of Medicine. 2001. *Coverage Matters: Insurance and Health Care*. Washington, DC: National Academy Press.

Institute of Medicine. 2002. *Health Insurance Is a Family Matter*. Washington, DC: National Academy Press.

Institute of Medicine. 2003a. *Hidden Costs, Value Lost: Uninsurance in America*. Washington, DC: National Academy Press.

Institute of Medicine. 2003b. *A Shared Destiny: Community Effects of Uninsurance*. Washington, DC: National Academy Press.

Jacoby, Melissa B., Teresa A. Sullivan, and Elizabeth Warren. 2001. "Rethinking the Debates over Health Care Financing: Evidence from the Bankruptcy Courts." *New York University Law Review* 76:375–418.

Juster, F. Thomas, and Richard Suzman. 1995. "An Overview of the Health and Retirement Study." *Journal of Human Resources* 30:S7–56.

Kaiser Family Foundation. 2008. *Employer Health Benefits 2008 Annual Survey*. pp. exhibit 1.2. Washington, DC: Kaiser Family Foundation.

Katz, Michael. 1990. *The Undeserving Poor: From the War on Poverty to the War on Welfare*. New York: Alfred A. Knopf.

Kennickell, Arthur B. 2006. *How Do We Know If We Aren't Looking? An Investigation of Data Quality in the 2004 SCF*. pp. 1–34. Seattle, WA: American Statistical Association.

Kitchener, Martin, Terence Ng, Micky Willmott, and Charlene Harrinton. 2006. *The Texas Medicaid State Plan Personal Care Services Program*. San Francisco, CA: Center for Personal Assistance Services, University of California.

Kochhar, Rakesh. 2005. *The Occupational Status and Mobility of Hispanics*. Washington, DC: Pew Hispanic Center.

Kochhar, Rakesh. 2008. "Latino Labor Report, 2008: Construction Reverses Job Growth for Latinos." in *Latino Labor Report*. Washington, DC: Pew Hispanic Center.

Kohler, Adriana D., and Melissa Lazarin. 2007. *Hispanic Education in the United States*. Washington, DC: National Council of la Raza.

Kymlicka, Will. 1995. *Multicultural Citizenship: A Liberal Theory of Minority Rights*. New York: Oxford University Press.

Kymlicka, Will. 2007. *Multiculatural Odysseys: Navigating the New International Politics of Diversity*. Oxford, England: Oxford University Press.

Kymlicka, Will, and Wayne Norman. 2000. "Citizenship in Culturally Diverse Societies: Issues, Contexts, Concepts." pp. 1–41 in *Citizenship in Diverse Societies*. Oxford and New York: Oxford University Press.

Ladd, Richard C., Robert L. Kane, Rosalie A. Kane, and Wendy J. Nielsen. 1995. *State LTC Profiles Report*. Minneapolis, MN: University of Minnesota.

Laise, Eleanor. 2009. "Big Slide in 401(k)s Spurs Calls for Change." in *The Wall Street Journal*. New York: Dow Jones & Company.

Landale, Nancy S., and R. S. Oropesa. 2007. "Hispanic Families: Stability and Change." *Annual Review of Sociology* 33:381–405.

Landale, Nancy S., R. Salvador Oropesa, and Cristina Bradatan. 2006. "Hispanic Families in the United States: Family Structure and Process in an Era of Family Change." pp. 138–178 in *Hispanics and the Future of America,* edited by Marta Tienda and Faith Mitchell. Washington, DC: National Academy Press.

Lazo, Alejandro. 2008. *Hispanics Hit Hard as Workers Lose Hours More Full-Time Jobs Turn Part-Time*. Washington, DC: The Washington Post Company.

Leland, John. 2009. "Downturn Puts a Chokehold on Those Caring for Family Members." pp. A16 in *New York Times*. New York: New York Times.

Lewin Group. 2004. *Actuarial Assessment of Medicaid Managed Care Expansion Options*. Austin, TX: Prepared for the Texas Health and Human Services Commission.

Lewis, Gail. 2005. "Welcome to the Margins: Diversity, Tolerance, and Policies of Exclusion." *Ethnic and Racial Studies* 28:536–558.

Lewis, Gail, and Sarah Neal. 2005. "Introduction: Contemporary Political Contexts, Changing Terrains and Revisited Discourses." *Ethnic and Racial Studies* 28:423–444.

Lewis, Oscar. 1959. *Five Families: Mexican Case Studies in the Culture of Poverty*. New York: New American Library.

Lewis, Oscar. 1966. *La Vida: A Puerto Rican Family in the Culture of Poverty – San Juan and New York*. New York: Random House.

Lichter, Daniel T., Deborah Roempke Graefe, and J. Brian Brown. 2003. "Is Marriage a Panacea? Union Formation Among Economically Disadvantaged Unwed Mothers." *Social Problems* 50:60–86.

Long, Bridget Terry, and Michal Kurlaender. 2008. *Do Community Colleges Provide a Viable Pathway to a Baccalaureate Degree?* Washington, DC: National Bureau of Economic Research.

Long, Sharon K., and Yu-Chu Shen. 2004. "Changing Options for Insurance Coverage: How Does the Future Look for Low- and Middle-Income Workers if Employer Sponsored Coverage Is Not an Option?" in *Health Policy On-Line, No. 10*. Washington, DC: The Urban Institute.

Lopez, Mark Hugo, and Michael T. Light. 2009. *A Rising Share: Hispanics and Federal Crime*. Washington, DC: Pew Hispanic Center.

Lowell, B. Lindsay, and Roberto Suro. 2002. *The Improving Educational Profile of Latino Immigrants*. Washington, DC: Pew Hispanic Center.

Lucas, Robert E. B. 2008. *International Labor Migration in a Globalizing Economy*. Washington, DC: Carnegie Endowment for International Peace.

Lupton, Joseph P., and James P. Smith. 2003. "Marriage, Assets, and Savings." pp. 129–152 in *Marriage and the Economy Theory and Evidence from Advanced Industrial Societies,* edited by Shoshana A. Grossbard-Shechtman. New York: Cambridge University Press.

Lusardi, Annamaria, and Olivia S. Mitchell. 2007. "Financial Literacy and Retirement Planning: Implications for Retirement Well Being." *Journal of Monetary Economics* 54:205–224.

Maag, Elaine. 2005. *Disparities in Knowledge of EITC*. Washington, DC: Urban Institute.

Manton, Kenneth G., and Eric Stallard. 1992. "Analysis of Underwriting Factors for AAPCC." *Health Care Financing Review* 14:117–132.

Markides, Kyriakos S., Laura Rudkin, Ronald J. Angel, and David Espino. 1997. "Health Status of Hispanic Elderly." pp. 285–300 in *Racial and Ethnic Differences in the Health of Older Americans,* edited by Linda G. Martin and Beth J. Soldo. Washington, DC: National Academy Press.

Marshall, T. H. 1950. *Citizenship and Social Class: And Other Essays.* Cambridge, England: Cambridge University Press.

Martin, Patricia P. 2007. *Hispanics, Social Security, and Supplement Security Income.* Baltimore, MC: Social Security Administration.

Matute-Bianchi, Maria Eugenia. 1986. "Ethnic Identities and Patterns of School Success and Failure among Mexican-Descent and Japanese-American Students in a California High School: An Ethnographic Analysis." *American Journal of Education* 95:233–255.

Mead, Lawrence M. 1986. *Beyond Entitlement.* New York: The Free Press.

Mead, Lawrence M. 1997. "Citizenship and Social Policy: T. H. Marshall and Poverty." *Social Philosophy and Policy* 14:197–230.

Medicare Rights Center. 2008. *What Is Not Covered by Medicare?* Washington, DC: Medicare Rights Center.

Ménard, Claude, and Mary M. Shirley (Eds.). 2005. *Handbook of New Institutional Economics.* Dordrecht, The Netherlands: Springer.

Meschede, Tatjana, Thomas M. Shapiro, and Jennifer Wheary. 2009. *Living Longer on Less: The New Economic (Insecurity) of Seniors.* Waltham, MA: The Institute on Assets and Social Policy, Brandeis University.

Metropolitan Life Insurance Company. 2005. "The Metlife Study of Employee Benefit Trends: 2004." in *Coping with Financially Dependent Parents, Hispanic Workers Worry About the Future.* New York.

Meyer, Madonna Harrington, and Pamela Herd. 2007. *Market Friendly or Family Friendly?: The State and Gender Inequality in Old Age.* New York: Russell Sage Foundation.

Mintz, S. 2007. "Mexican Americans and the New Deal." *Digital History.* www.digtalhistory.

Misra, Joya. 1999. "Latinas and African American Women in the Labor Market: Implications for Policy." pp. 408–431 in *Latinas and African-American Women at Work,* edited by Irene Browne. New York: Russell Sage Foundation.

Montez, Jennifer Karas, Jacqueline L. Angel, and Ronald J. Angel. 2009. "Work and Family Sources of Inequality in Health Care Coverage for Mexican-Origin Women." *Journal of Health and Social Behavior* 50:132–148.

Moen, Phyllis, and Patricia Roehling. 2004. *The Career Mystique: Cracks in the American Dream. Lanham:* Rowman & Littlefield Publishers, Inc.

Moon, Marilyn, and Pamela Herd. 2003. *A Report on Women's Needs and Medicare Reform.* New York: The Century Foundation Press.

Montes de Oca, Verónica, Ahtziri Molina, and Rosaura Avalos. 2008. *Migración, redes transnacionales y envejecimiento: Estudio de las redes familiares transnacionales de la vejez en Guanajuato.* Mexico, D.F.: Universidad Nacional Autónoma de México, Instituto de Investigaciones Sociales, Gobierno Del Estado de Guanajuato.

Moreno, Susan E., and Chandra Muller. 1996. "Lantinas in the U.S. Labor Force." pp. 38–41 in *Women and Work,* edited by Paula J. Dubeck and Kathryn Borman. New York: Garland Publishing, Inc.

Mumola, Christopher J. 2000. *Incarcerated Parents and Their Children.* Washington, DC: Bureau of Justice Statistics.

Munnell, Alicia H., and Annika Sundén. 2004. *Coming Up Short: The Challenge of 401(k) Plans.* Washington, DC: Brookings Institution.

Murdock, Steve H., Steve White, Md. Nazrul Hoque, Beverly Pecotte, Xiuhong You, and Jennifer Balkan. 2002. *The Texas Challenge in the Twenty-First Century: Implications of Population Change for the Future of Texas.* San Antonio, TX: Institute for Demographic and Socioeconomic Research, The University of Texas at San Antonio.

Murguía, Janet. 2007. *Earned Income Tax Credit Outreach*. Washington, DC: National Council of La Raza.
Murray, Charles. 1994. *Losing Ground: American Social Policy 1950–1980*. New York: Basic Books.
Murray, Charles. 1996. "Charles Murray and the Underclass: The Developing Debate." in *Choice in Welfare No. 33*. London, England: The IEA Health and Welfare Unit.
Murray, Charles. 1999. *The Underclass Revisited*. Washington, DC: AEI Press.
Murray, Charles. 2006. *In Our Hands: A Plan to Replace the Welfare State*. Blue Ridge Summit, PA: AEI Press.
Myles, John. 1984. *Old Age in the Welfare State: The Political Economy of Public Pensions*. Boston, MA: Little Brown.
National Bureau of Economic Research. 2004. *Social Security and Elderly Poverty*. Cambridge, MA: National Bureau of Economic Research.
National Center for Education Statistics. 2004. *High School Graduates Who Completed Advanced Science and Mathematics Courses in 2000 by Race and Ethnicity*. Washington, DC: U.S. Department of Education.
National Center for Education Statistics. 2005. *Number and Percentage Distribution of Degrees Conferred by Degree-granting Institutions, by Level of Degree, Race/ethnicity, and Sex: 2003–04*. Washington, DC: U.S. Department of Education.
National Center for Education Statistics. 2007c. *First-Professional Degrees Conferred by Degree-Granting Institutions in Dentistry, Medicine, and Law, by Number of Institutions Conferring Degrees and Sex of Student: Selected Years, 1949–50 Through 2005–06*, Washington, DC: U.S. Department of Education.
National Center for Education Statistics. 2007a. *Percentage of Persons Age 25 and Over and 25 to 29, By Race/Ethnicity, Years of School Completed, and Sex: Selected Years, 1910 Through 2007*. Washington, DC: U.S. Department of Education.
National Center for Education Statistics. 2007b. *Table 26.2. Number and Percentage of Persons Age 25 to 29 with Bachelor's Degree or Higher, By Race/Ethnicity with Hispanic and Asian Subgroups: 2005*, edited by Status and Trends in the Education of Racial and Ethnic Minorities. Washington, DC: U.S. Department of Eduation, Institute of Education Sciences.
National Council of La Raza. 2000. *Hispanics and the Earned Income Tax Credit*. Washington, DC.
National Council of La Raza. 2004. *Pension Coverage: A Missing Step in the Wealth-Building Ladder for Latinos*. Washington, DC: National Council of La Raza.
National Council of La Raza. 2005a. *Retirement Security for Latinos: Bolstering Coverage, Savings, and Adequacy*. Washington, DC: The Retirement Security Project.
National Council of La Raza. 2005b. *The Social Security Program and Reform: The Latino Perspective*. Washington, DC.
National Council of La Raza. 2008. "Medicaid and SCHIP: Critical for Latino Families Facing Financial Hardship." in *NCLF Fact Sheet*. Washington, DC: National Council of La Raza.
Navarrette, Ruben. 2009. "Hispanics in U.S. Senate Endangered." in *The Latino Journal*. Sacramento, CA: Latino Journal Blogspot.
Noble, Charles. 1997. *Welfare as We Knew It*. Oxford, Eng.: Oxford University Press.
Oberlander, Jonathan. 2001. "Political Analysis and Medical Care: The Politics of Medicare Reconsidered." *Journal of Health Politics, Policy and Law* 26:139–146.
Montes de Oca, Verónica, Ahtziri Molina, and Rosaura Avalos. 2008. *Migración, redes transnacionales y envejecimiento: Estudio de las redes familiares transnacionales de la vejez en Guanajuato*. Mexico, DF: Universidad Nacional Autónoma de México, Instituto de Investigaciones Sociales, Gobierno Del Estado de Guanajuato.
O'Connor, Alice. 2002. *Poverty Knowledge: Social Science, Social Policy, and the Poor in Twentieth-Century U.S. History*. Princeton, NJ: Princeton University Press.
Orloff, Ann Shola. 1993. "Gender and the Social Rights of Citizenship: State Policies and Gender Relations in Comparative Research." *American Sociological Review* 58:303–328.

Oropesa, R. S. 1996. "Normative Beliefs About Marriage and Cohabitation: A Comparison of Non-Latino Whites, Mexican Americans, and Puerto Ricans." *Journal of Marriage and Family* 58:49–62.

Orszag, Peter R., and Eric Rodriguez. 2005. *Retirement Security for Latinos: Bolstering Coverage, Savings, and Adequacy*. Washington, DC: The Retirement Security Project, National Council of La Raza.

Passel, Jeffrey S., and D'Vera Cohn. 2008. *U.S. Population Projections: 2005–2050*. Washington, DC: Pew Research Center.

Pascall, Gillian, and Jane Lewis. 2004. "Emerging Gender Regimes and Policies for Gender Equality in a Wider Europe." *Journal of Social Policy* 33:373–394.

Perlmann, Joel, and Roger Waldinger. 1997. "Second Generation Decline? Immigrant Children Past and Present – A reconsideration." *International Migration Review* 31:893–922.

Perry, Michael, Susan Kannel, R. Burciaga Valdez, and Christina Chang. 2000. "Medicaid and Children: Overcoming Barriers to Enrollment." in *The Kaiser Commission on Medicaid and the Uninsured: Findings from a National Survey*. Washington, DC: Henry J. Kaiser Family Foundation.

Pew Hispanic Center. 2006. *Households by Income, Race, and Ethnicity: 2006*, edited by Statistical Portrait of Hispanics in the United States. Washington, DC: Pew Hispanic Center.

Pew Hispanic Center. 2008. *Statistical Portrait of Hispanics in the United States, 2006*. Washington, DC: The Pew Charitable Trusts.

Phillips, Katherin Ross. 2001. "Who Knows about the Earned Income Tax Credit?" in *New Federalism: National Survey of America's Families*. Washington, DC: The Urban Institute.

Pierson, Paul. 2001a. "Coping with Permanent Austerity: Welfare State Restructuring in Affluent Democracies." pp. 410–456 in *The New Politics of the Welfare State*, edited by Pau Pierson. Oxford and New York: Oxford University Press.

Pierson, Paul. 2001b. "Post-Industrial Pressures on the Mature Welfare States." pp. 80–106 in *The New Politics of the Welfare State*, edited by Paul Pierson. Oxford, Eng. and New York: Oxford University Press.

Pierson, Paul. 2004. *Politics in Time: History, Institutions, and Social Analysis*. Princeton, NJ: Princeton University Press.

Pino, Diana Marie. 2005. "Persistence of First-Generation Mexican American University Students in a Hispanic Serving Institution." in *College of Education*. Austin, TX: University of Texas at Austin.

Poole, Mary. 2006. *The Segregated Origins of Social Security: African Americans and the Welfare State*. Chapel Hill, NC: University of North Carolina Press.

Portes, Alejandro, and Robert Bach. 1985. *Latin Journey: Cuban and Mexican Immigrants in the United States*. Berkeley, CA: University of California Press.

Portes, Alejandro, Patricia Fernández-Kelly, and William Haller. 2005. "Segmented Assimilation on the Ground: The New Second Generation in Early Adulthood." *Ethnic and Racial Studies* 28:1000–1040.

Portes, Alejandro, and Rubén Rumbaut. 2001. *Legacies: The Story of the Immigrant Second Generation*. Berkeley, CA: University of California Press and Russell Sage Foundation.

Portes, Alejandro, and Rubén G. Rumbaut. 1996. *Immigrant America: A Portrait*. Berkeley, CA: University of California Press.

Portes, Alejandro, and Rubén G. Rumbaut. 2006. *Immigrant America: A Portrait*. Berkeley, CA: University of California Press.

Portes, Alejandro, and Min Zhou. 1993. "The New Second Generation: Segmented Assimilation and Its Variants." *The Annals of the American Academy of Political and Social Science* 530: 74–96.

Portes, Pedro R. 1999. "Social and Psychological Factors in the Academic Achievement of Children of Immigrants: A Cultural History Puzzle." *American Educational Research Journal* 36:489–507.

Poulat, Emile. 2003. *Notre Laïcité Publique*. Paris: Berg International Editeurs.

Princeton Survey Research Associates, American Families Discuss Social Security Project. 1998. *Hispanic Attitudes Toward Social Security*. Washington, DC: The Pew Research Center.

Quadagno, Jill. 2004. "Why the United States Has No National Health Insurance: Stakekholder Mobilization Against the Welfare State: 1945–1996." *Journal of Health and Social Behavior* 45:25–44.

Quadagno, Jill. 1988a. "From Old-Age Assistance to Supplemental Security Income: The Political Economy of Relief in the South, 1935–1972." in *The Politics of Social Policy in the United States*, edited by Margaret Weir, Ann Shola Orloff, and Theda Skocpol. Princeton, NJ: Princeton University Press.

Quadagno, Jill. 1988b. *The Transformation of Old Age Security: Class and Politics in the American Welfare State*. Chicago, IL: University of Chicago Press.

Quadagno, Jill. 1994. *The Color of Welfare: How Racism Undermined the War on Poverty*. New York, Oxford: Oxford University Press.

Quadagno, Jill. 2005. *One Nation, Uninsured: Why the U.S. Has No National Health Insurance*. New York, Oxford: Oxford University Press.

Quadagno, Jill, and Debra Street. 2006. "New Directions in U.S. Welfare State Policy: Minor Retrenchment or Major Transformation?" *Research on Aging* 28:1–14.

Quinn, Kevin. 2000. *Working Without Benefits: The Health Insurance Crisis Confronting Hispanic Americans*. Washington, DC: Kaiser Commission on Medicaid and the Uninsured.

Raley, Kelly R., T. Elizabeth Durden, and Elizabeth Wildsmith. 2004. "Understanding Mexican-American Marriage Patterns Using a Life-Course Approach." *Social Science Quarterly* 85:872–890.

Ramirez, Roberto R. 2004. *We the People: Hispanic in the United States. Census 2000 Special Report* p 20–545. Washington, DC: U.S. Census Bureau.

Ramirez, Roberto R., and G. Patricia de la Cruz. 2003. "The Hispanic Population in the United States: March 2002." in *Current Population Reports*. p 20–545 Washington, DC: U.S. Census Bureau.

Reich, Robert B. 2007. *Supercapitalism: The Transformation of Business, Democracy, and Everyday Life*. New York: Alfred A. Knopf.

Reimers, Cornelia. 2006. "Economic Well-Being." pp. 291–361 in *Hispanics and the Future of America*, edited by Marta Tienda and Faith Mitchell. Washington, DC: National Academies Press.

Romano, Flavio. 2006. *Clinton and Blair: The Political Economy of the Third Way*. New York: Routledge.

Romo, Harriett D., and Toni Falbo. 1996. *Latino High School Graduation: Defying the Odds*. Austin, TX: University of Texas Press.

Rudolph, Noemi V., and James Lubitz. 1999. "Capitated Payment Approaches for Medicaid-Financed Long-term Care." *Health Care Financing Review* 21:51–64.

Santos, Roberto, and Patricia Seitz. 2000. "Benefit Coverage for Latino and Latina Workers." pp. 162–185 in *Moving Up the Economic Ladder: Latino Workers and the Nation's Future Prosperity*, edited by Sonia M. Perez. Washington, DC: National Council of La Raza.

Sanzenbacher, Geoffrey. 2006. *Estimating Pension Coverage Using Different Data Sets*. Chestnut Hill, MA: Center for Retirement Research, Boston College.

Schierup, Carl-Ulrik, Peo Hansen, and Stephen Castels. 2006. *Migration, Citizenship, and the European Welfare State: A European Dilemma*. Oxford, England: Oxford University Press.

Schlesinger, Arthur Jr. 1992. *The Disuniting of America*. New York: Norton.

Schoen, Cathy, Patricia Neuman, Michellel Kitchman, Karen Davis, and Diane Rowland. 1998. *Medicare Beneficiaries: A Population at Risk, Commonwealth Fund*. New York: Commonwealth Fund.

Schulz, James, and Robert Binstock. 2006. *Aging Nation: The Economics and Politics of Growing Older in America*. Westport, CT: Praeger Publishers.

Schur, Claudia L., L. A. Albers, and Marc L. Berk. 1995. "Health Care Use by Hispanic Adults: Financial vs. Non-financial Determinants." *Health Care Financing Review* 17:71–88.

Schur, Claudia L., and Jacob Feldman. 2000. *Running in Place: How Job Characteristics, Immigrant Status, and Family Structure Keep Hispanics Uninsured*. New York: The Commonwealth Fund.

Schwarz, Karen, Catherine Hoffman, and Allison Cook. 2007 *Health Insurance Coverage of America's Children*. Washington, DC: Kaiser Commission on Medicaid and the Uninsured, The Henry J. Kaiser Family Foundation.

Selden, Thomas M., Jessica S. Banthin, and Joel W. Cohen. 1998. "Medicaid's Problem Children: Eligible but Not Enrolled." *Health Affairs* 17:192–200.

Sevak, Purvi, David R. Weir, and Robert J. Willis. 2003–2004. "The Economic Consequences of a Husband's Death: Evidence from the HRS and AHEAD." in *Social Security Bulletin*. Baltimore, MD: Social Security Administration.

Shefner, Jon. 2008. *The Illusion of Civil Society: Democratization and Community Mobilization in Low-Income Mexico*. University Park, PA: The Pennsylvania State University Press.

Shen, Yu-Chu, and Steven Zuckerman. 2003. "Why Is There State Variation in Employer-Sponsored Insurance?" *Health Affairs* 22:24–151.

Short, Pamela Farley. 1998. "Gaps and Transitions in Health Insurance: What Are the Concerns of Women?" *Journal of Women's Health* 7:725–737.

Shuey, Kim M., and Andrea E. Willson. 2008. "Cumulative Disadvantage and Black/White Differences in Life Course Health Trajectories." *Research on Aging* 30:220–225.

Sigerist, Henry E. 1999. "From Bismarck to Beveridge: Developments and Trends in Social Security Legislation." *Journal of Public Health Policy* 20:474–496.

Smeeding, Timothy M. 2000. "Changing Income Inequality in OECD Countries: Updated Results from the Luxembourg Income Study (LIS)." in *The Personal Distribution of Income in an International Perspective*, edited by Richard Hauser and Irene Becker. Berlin: Springer-Verlag.

Smeeding, Timothy M., Lee Rainwater, and Gray Burtless. 2001. "U.S. Poverty in a Cross-National Context." pp. 162–189 in *Understanding Poverty*, edited by Sheldon H. Danziger and Robert H. Haveman. New York and Cambridge, MA: Russell Sage Foundation and Harvard University Press.

Smith, Dayle M. 2000. *Women at Work: Leadership for the Next Century*. Saddle River, NJ: Prentice Hall.

Smith, James P., and Barry Edmonston. 1997. *The New Americans: Economic, Demographic, and Fiscal Effects of Immigration*. Washington, DC: National Academcy Press.

Smith, Vernon K., and David M. Rousseau. 2005. *SCHIP Enrollment in 50 States: December 2004 Data Update*. Washington, DC: The Kaiser Commission on Medicaid and the Uninsured.

Social Security Administration. 2000. "By Marital Status, Sex of Nonmarried Persons, Race, and Hispanic Origin." Table 7.4 in *Social Security Administration*, 2000: Shares of Aggregate Income of the Population 55 or Older, by Source. Baltimore, MD: Social Security Administration.

Social Security Administration. 2004a. *The 2004 Annual Report of the Board of Trustees of the Federal Old-Age and Survivors Insurance and Disability Insurance Trust Fund, Table IV.B2*. Washington, DC: The Social Security Administration.

Social Security Administration. 2004b. "Covered Workers and Beneficiaries, Calendar Years 1945–2080" pp. Table IV.B2 in *The 2004 Annual Report of the Board of Trustees of the Federal Old-Age and Survivors Insurance and Disability Insurance Trust Fund*. Baltimore, MD: Social Security Administration.

Social Security Administration. 2005. *Income of the Population 55 or Older: 2002*. Baltimore, MD: Social Security Administration.

Social Security Administration. 2009. "Statements Giving Reasons Why Certain Groups Were Excluded from Social Security Act." pp. 112–113 in *Social Security History*. Baltimore, MD: Social Security Administration.

Spain, Daphne, and Suzanne M. Bianchi. 1996. *Balancing Act: Motherhood, Marriage, and Employment Among American Women*. New York: Russell Sage Foundation.

Starr, Paul. 1982. *The Transformation of American Medicine: The Rise of a Soverign Profession and the Making of a Vast Industry*. New York: Basic Books.

Stevens, Beth. 1988. "Blurring the Boundaries: How the Federal Government Has Influenced Welfare Benefits in the Private Sector." in *The Politics of Social Policy in the United States*, edited by Margaret Weir, Ann Shola Orloff, and Theda Skocpol. Princeton, NJ: Princeton University Press.

Stevenson, David, Brian Burwell, and Michael Schaefer. 2006. *The Nursing Home Liability Insurance Market: A Case Study of Texas*. Washington, DC: U.S. Department of Health and Human Services.

Stockton, John, Ray Bryant, and Liliana Santoyo. 2001. *Enrollment of Hispanic Dual Eligibles on the Texas-Mexico Border*. Austin, TX: Texas Department of Human Services, Office of Aging Policy and Information, Texas Department on Aging.

Stoddard, Scott. 2008. "Workers Giving Up and Part-Time Jobs Mask Labor Woes." *Investor's Business Daily*. www.investors.com

Stolzenberg, Ross M. 1990. "Ethnicity, Geography, and Occupational Achievement of Hispanic Men in the United States." *American Sociological Review* 55:143–154.

Suárez-Orozco, Marcelo M., and Carola Suárez-Orozco. 1995. "The Cultural Patterning of Achievement Motivation: A Comparative Study of Mexican, Mexican Immigrant, and Non-Latino White American Youth in Schools." pp. 161–190 in *California's Immigrant Children: Theory, Research, and Implications for Educational Policy*, edited by Robén G. Rumbaut and Wayne A. Cornelius. San Diego, CA: La Jolla, Center for U.S.-Mexican Studies, University of California.

Suro, Roberto, and Audrey Singer. 2002. *Latino Growth in Metropolitan America: Changing Patterns*. Washington, DC: The Brookings Institution.

Survey of Consumer Finances. 2007. Washington, DC: The Federal Reserve Board, U.S. Department of the Treasury.

Swank, Duane. 2001. "Political Institutions and Welfare State Restructuring: The Impact of Institutions on Social Policy Change in Developed Democracies." pp. 197–237 in *The New Politics of the Welfare State*, edited by Paul Pierson. Oxford, Eng. and New York: Oxford University Press.

Tanner, Michael. 2005. "Individual Free Liberty, Markets, and Peace." in *Committee on Ways and Means, Subcommittee on Social Security*. Washington, DC: Cato Institute, Project on Social Security Choice.

Taylor, Charles. 1994. "The Politics of Recognition." pp. 25–73 in *Multiculturalism: Examining the Politics of Recognition*, edited by Amy Gutman. Princeton, NJ: Princeton University Press.

Telles, Edward E., and Vilma Ortiz. 2008. *Generations of Exclusion: Mexican Americans, Assimilation, and Race*. New York: Russell Sage Foundation.

Texas Department of Aging. 2003. *Texas Demograpics: Older Adults in Texas*. Austin, TX: Office of Aging Policy and Information.

Texas Department on Aging. 2002. *Older Adult Profile: Hispanics in Texas*. Austin, TX: Office of Aging Policy and Information.

Texas House of Representatives. 2005. *State Finance Report: The House Appropriations Committee's Proposed Budget for Fiscal 2006–07*. Austin, TX: House Research Organization.

Texas State Data Center. 2006. *Summary of Trends in Texas State Data Center 2006: Population Projections*. San Antonio, TX: University of Texas Health Science Center.

The Association for the Advancement of Mexican Americans. 2009. *AAMA Educational Programs*. Houston, TX: The Association for the Advancement of Mexican Americans.

Thomas, Duncan, V. Joseph Hotz, and Stephen J. Trejo. 2006. *Hispanics and the Future of America*. pp. 228–290. Washington, DC: National Academies Press.

Tienda, Marta. 2007. "Hispanics at the Age Crossroads: Opportunities and Risks." *Focus Spring-Summer*: 27–32.

Tienda, Marta, and Faith Mitchell. 2006a. *Hispanics and the Future of America*. Washington, DC: National Academy Press.

Tienda, Marta, and Faith Mitchell (Eds.). 2006b. *Multiple Origins, Uncertain Destinies: Hispanics and the American Future*. Washington, DC: The National Academy Press.

Torres-Gil, Fernando, Robert Greenstein, and David Kamin. 2005. *The Importance of Social Security to the Hispanic Community*. Washington, DC: Center on Budget and Policy Priorities.

Toussaint-Comeau, Maude. 2004. *The Occupational Assimilation of Hispanics in the U.S.: Evidence from Panel Data*. Chicago, IL: Federal Reserve Bank of Chicago.

Treviño, Fernando M., M. Eugene Moyer, R. Burciaga Valdez, and Christine A. Stroup-Benham. 1991. "The Health Insurance Coverage of Hispanics." *Journal of the American Medical Association* 265:233–237.

Tritz, Karen. 2005. Dual Eligibles. in *A CRS Series on Medicaid*. Washington, DC: Congressional Research Service, Library of Congress.

Tussie, Dianna, Marcos Mendiburu, and Patricia Vázques. 1997. "Los nuevos mandatos de los Bancos Multilaterales de Desarrollo: su aplicación al caso de Argentina." in *El BID, el Banco Mundial y la sociedad civil : nuevas modalidades de financiamiento internacional*, edited by Diana Tussie. Buenos Aires, Argentina: Oficina de Publicaciones del CBC, Universidad de Buenos Aires, Facultad Latinoamericana de Ciencias Sociales.

U.S. Census Bureau. 2002. *Current Population Survey: Design and Methodology. Technical Paper 63RV*. Washington, DC: Government Printing Office.

U.S. Census Bureau. 2003. "Cities with 250,000 or More Inhabitants in 2000 – Hispanic and Non-Hispanic Groups: 2000." pp. Table 33 in *Statistical Abstract of the United States: 2003*. Washington, DC: Government Printing Office.

U.S. Census Bureau. 2005. "Income Stable, Poverty Up, Numbers of Americans With and Without Health Insurance Rise." *International Journal of Health Servicies* 35:117–124.

U.S. Census Bureau. 2006a. *Current Population Survey, 2006 Annual Social and Economic (ASEC) Supplement*. Retrieved May 6, 2007 (http://www.census.gov/apsd/techdoc/-cps/cpsmar06.pdf).

U.S. Census Bureau. 2006b. *Table 1: Annual Estimates of the Population for Incorporated Places Over 100,000, Ranked by July 1, 2006 Population: April 1, 2000 to July 1, 2006*. Washington, DC: U.S. Department of Commerce.

U.S. Census Bureau. 2008a. *2008 National Population Projections: Projections of the Population by Sex, Race, and Hispanic Origin for the United States: 2010 to 2050*. Washington, DC: U.S. Department of Commerce.

U.S. Census Bureau. 2008b. "Family Groups with Children Under 18 Years Old by Race and Hispanic Origin: 1990 to 2007." *Current Population Reports, P20-537*. Washington, DC: U.S. Department of Commerce.

U.S. Census Bureau Census Bureau. 2009. "Nation's Population Growing Older, More Diverse." Washington, DC: U.S. Census Bureau.

U.S. Department of Labor. 2005. *Women in the Labor Force: A Data Book*. Washington, DC: U.S. Department of Labor.

U.S. Office of Personnel Management, The Federal Long-Term Care Insurance Program. 2008. *Find the Cost of Care in Your Area*. Washington, DC: U.S. Office of Personnel Management.

Valadez, Jorge M. 2001. *Deliberative Democracy, Political Legitimacy, and Self-Determination in Multicultural Societies*. Boulder, CO: Westview Press.

Vandello, Joseph, and Dov Cohen. 2003. "Male Honor and Female Fidelity: Implicit Cultural Scripts that Perpetuate Domestic Violence." *Journal of Personality and Social Psychology* 84:997–1010.

Waldron, Ingrid, Mary Elizabeth Hughes, and Tracy L. Brooks. 1996. "Marriage Protection and Marriage Selection – Prospective Evidence for Reciprocal Effects of Marital Status and Health." *Social Science & Medicine* 43:113–123.

Waldron, Ingrid, Christopher C. Weiss, and Mary Elizabeth Hughes. 1998. "Interacting Effects of Multiple Roles on Women's Health." *Journal of Health and Social Behavior* 39:216–236.

Wallace, Steven P. 2007. *Immigration, Health and Work: The Facts Behind the Myths*. Los Angeles, CA: University of California, Los Angeles.

Weinberg, David H. 2004. "Evidence from Census 2000 about Earnings by Detailed Occupation for Men and Women." in *Census 2000 Special Reports CENSR-15*. Washington, DC: U.S. Census Bureau.

Weir, Margaret, Ann Shola Orloff, and Theda Skocpol (Eds.). 1988. *The Politics of Social Policy in the United States*. Princeton, NJ: Princeton University Press.

Willson, Andrea E. 2003. "Race and Women's Income Trajectories: Employment, Marriage, and Income Security Over the Life Course." *Social Problems* 50:87–110.

Wilson, William J. 1987. *The Truly Disadvantaged: The Inner City, The Underclass, and Public Policy*. Chicago, IL: University of Chicago Press.

Wilson, William Julius. 1996. *When Work Disappears: The World of the Urban Poor*. New York: Knopf.

Wilson, William Julius. 2009. *More Than Just Race: Being Black and Poor in the Inner City*. New York: W.W. Norton.

Winston, Pamela, Ronald J. Angel, Linda M. Burton, Lindsay Chase-Lansdale, Andrew J. Cherlin, Robert A. Moffitt, and William Julius Wilson. 1999. *Welfare, Children, and Families: A Three-City Study, Overview and Design*. Baltimore, MD: Johns Hopkins University.

Wojtkiewicz, Roger A., and Katherine M. Donato. 1995. "Hispanic Educational Attainment: the Effects of Family Background and Nativity." *Social Forces* 74:559–574.

Wood, Robert G., Brian Goesling, Sarah Avellar, and Mathematica Policy Research Incorporated. 2007. *The Effects of Marriage on Health: A Synthesis of Recent Research Evidence*. Washington, DC: Office of the Assistant Secretary for Planning and Evaluation, U.S. Department of Health and Human Services.

Yoon, Young-Hee. 1996. "Intersection of Gender, Race/Ethnicity, and Work." pp. 35–38 in *Women and Work*, edited by Paula J. Dubeck and Kathryn Borman. New York: Garland Publishing Inc.

Zambrana, Ruth E., and Laura A. Logie. 2000. "Latino Child Health: Need for Inclusion in National Discourse." *American Journal of Public Health* 90:1827–1833.

Zuberi, Dan. 2006. *Differences that Matter: Social Policy and the Working Poor in the United States and Canada*. Ithaca, NY and London: Cornell University Press.

Subject Index

Note: The letters ‘f’ and ‘t’ following the locators refer to figures and tables respectively.

LaVergne, TN USA
11 September 2009

157354LV00002BB/2/P

9 781441 904737